LPN
to RN
Transitions

LPN to RN Transitions

Lora Claywell, MSN, RN
St. Louis, Missouri

Bradley S. Corbin, MSN, RN
Education Specialist
Summerlin Hospital Medical Center
Las Vegas, Nevada

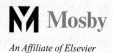
An Affiliate of Elsevier

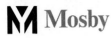

An Affiliate of Elsevier

11830 Westline Industrial Drive
St. Louis, Missouri 63146

NOTICE

Health care is an ever-changing field. Standard safety precautions must be followed, but as new research and clinical experience broaden our knowledge, changes in treatment and drug therapy may become necessary or appropriate. Readers are advised to check the most current product information provided by the manufacturer of each drug to be administered to verify the recommended dose, the method and duration of administration, and contraindications. It is the responsibility of the licensed prescriber, relying on experience and knowledge of the patient, to determine dosages and the best treatment for each individual patient. Neither the publisher nor the author assumes any liability for any injury and/or damage to persons or property arising from this publication.

Library of Congress Cataloging-in-Publication Data

Claywell, Lora
    LPN to RN transitions/Lora Claywell, Bradley S. Corbin.
      p.; cm.
    Includes bibliographical references and index.
      ISBN-13: 978-0-323-01091-7   ISBN-10: 0-323-01091-1 (softcover)
      1. Nursing—Vocational guidance. 2. Practical nurses. I. Title: Licensed Practical Nurse to Registered Nurse transitions. II. Corbin, Bradley S. III. Title.
      [DNLM: 1. Education, Nursing. 2. Career Mobility. 3. Nurse's Role. 4. Nursing Process.
    WY 18 C6225L 2003]
    RT82.C552 2003
    610.73'06'9—dc21   2002033770

Vice President and Publishing Director, Nursing: Sally Schrefer
Executive Editor: Michael S. Ledbetter
Associate Developmental Editor: Amanda Sunderman Politte
Publishing Services Manager: Catherine Jackson
Project Manager: Jeff Patterson
Designer: Teresa Breckwoldt

ISBN-13: 978-0-323-01091-7
ISBN-10: 0-323-01091-1

CE/MVY

Printed in the United States of America

Last digit is the print number: 9 8 7 6 5 4 3

Consultants

Martha S. Barnas, RN, MSN, MSEd
Professor, Program Head
Nursing
Virginia Western Community
 College
Roanoke, Virginia

Julie Barry, RN, PhD
Department of Health Sciences
John Wood Community College
Quincy, Illinois

Linda A. Earle, BS, BSN, MSN, RN, C
Adjunct Nursing Instructor
Associate Degree Nursing Program
Central Maine Technical College
Auburn, Maine

Brenda Hempen, RN
Coordinator, Nursing Education
Natural and Health Sciences
Hawkeye Community College
Waterloo, Iowa

Joyce T. Humphries, RN, MS
Coordinator
LPN Program
Rogue Community College
Grants Pass, Oregon

Dorothy Bell John, RN, MN
Assistant Professor
School of Nursing
University of Louisiana at Monroe
Monroe, Louisiana

Linda Rickabaugh, MSN, RN
Associate Professor
Faculty, Associate Degree Nursing
College of Health Sciences
Roanoke, Virginia

Clara B. Wallace, MN, RN
Instructor
School of Professional Nursing
Baptist Health System
San Antonio, Texas

Melissa T. Williams
Assistant Professor
Nursing
Augusta State University
Augusta, Georgia

Ann M.L. Woodward
Professor
Nursing
Kirkwood Community College
Cedar Rapids, Iowa

Acknowledgments

Our first thanks go to the courageous students who embark upon the journey of transition from LPN to RN. (It is not for the faint of heart.) You inspired the work, and this book is written for you. Many thanks go to the very patient and supportive staff at Mosby. To our reviewers whose careful read and thoughtful comments made a world of difference, thank you.

From Lora: I wish to thank my husband and best friend, Jim, and my wonderful children, Cameron and Kaitlin, for their unconditional love and enduring patience. You are my greatest source of joy and inspiration. You have sacrificed much so that I might make a difference. This work would not have been possible without your support. You are the lights of my life. I love you.

I wish also to thank my mom and dad, John and Grace Dunshee. Your influences continue to shine through in my life and in my work. I love you.

Thanks also to my brother John, his wife Chris, and their children. You're a great cheering section. Thank you for being there. I love you.

To Brad, my co-author, thank you for your dedication to our work. May you continue to feel inspired and know that your work is important.

From Brad: I want to recognize my son, Matt, who watched and encouraged me from afar. I gained strength in knowing that while I was working on my textbook, he was working on his own growth through life experiences. To my sister who believed in me even when I had doubts. To my mother who always had words of encouragement, never criticism. To my colleagues: I did it.

To Lora, my co-author, I found an individual who, with intellect and grace, was able to juggle a family, a career, and a scholarly quest with the demands and deadlines of writing a textbook. I have the greatest respect and admiration for you.

Preface

The concept for this book originated from our experiences with having to assign students many different textbooks in order to cover the content that is necessary to prepare the LPN to re-enter the student role and ultimately transition to the role of RN. The expense and inconvenience that necessarily accompanies a backpack full of books was an added burden to our already overtaxed adult students.

The topics were carefully selected based on years of trial and error with putting together the right recipe of material that best supports our students, particularly during formal transition courses. Concepts defined and explored within the book are intended to support and nurture the growth needed for the transition of the LPN to the new role as an RN.

The book is divided into two major parts. Part One, Transitioning to the Student Role, was created for the person considering returning to a nursing program or who is enrolled in his or her first course. Section 1, Understanding Yourself, includes three chapters aimed at assisting the student to honestly assess who and where he or she is in life. From this a solid plan is created to help the student build on gifts or strengths and neutralize barriers or weaknesses.

Section 2, Becoming a Successful Student, includes three chapters with a common goal—improving the likelihood of success as a student. Adults returning to a formal learning situation need to establish study habits to support their other efforts. Another skill that students need to develop is that of accessing and arranging support for their return to college. We have found that students need a great deal of encouragement when it comes to financing their education. Repeat to your students our mantra. "Never let lack of money hold you back. You can come up with what you need." Many students have related that this was important to hear.

Included at the end of Section 2 is a basic math review. We know very few people, in all levels of nursing, who do not need a solid refresher in this area. LPNs have learned what they need to pass medications in their current roles. However, medication calculation becomes increasingly complex in registered nursing, and a solid mathematical foundation is absolutely critical. We hope the early placement of the math chapter in this book will encourage early assessment of and practice with math skills.

Part Two, Transitioning to the Registered Nurse Role, is directed toward the student engaged in an RN program. The emphasis is on differentiating the roles of LPN and RN. While Section 3, Understanding the Difference Between LPN and RN, has the greatest concentration of role comparison, the differentiation continues as a thread throughout the rest of the book in an effort to encourage the LPN to continually consider how his or her practice will change and expand as he or she begins to take on the role of RN.

Section 4, Care Planner versus Care Giver: Distinguishing the Roles, is composed of seven chapters that specifically distinguish the major roles of the RN. This information is imparted early on to students who are currently practicing as LPNs because they will be actively observing RN practice, albeit unidimensionally. Often the complexity and depth of the RN role is obscured from the LPN perspective. This complexity becomes a source of role strain as the LPN juggles what he or she believes the role to be with what it is actually becoming.

Section 5, Role Differences in Managing the Consumer: The Health-Illness Continuum, is directed toward the student who is nearing completion of their RN program. Consumer perspectives about health and illness and differentiation of the primary, secondary, and tertiary practice settings are explored. The student is invited to create a plan for continuation of his or her journey. Final stages of role transition begin with the completion of the RN program. A plan will hopefully help the student continue the life-long quest for learning.

Completing the book, the Appendixes include tools and references we hope you will find useful throughout your nursing program and beyond. Our desire is that this text will not only benefit the nurse during the formal transition courses often found at the beginning of nursing programs, but will continue to serve the nurse well for years.

Contents

Part Two • Transitioning to the Registered Nurse Role

LPN to RN Transitions

Section 1

Understanding Yourself

Chapter 1

Past, Present, and Future: Assessing Your Accomplishments

Key Terms

cohort
experiential resume
long-term goal
moving
outcome priority
refreezing
scheme
short-term goal
unfreezing

Overview

In this chapter you will begin to assess yourself closely and prepare for your nursing education experience. In doing so you will consider why you believe you want to be a registered nurse (RN). You will review the positive and negative aspects of your past. You will look closely at the present, set goals, and chart your course into your future as an RN.

Where It All Begins

As an LPN returning to nursing school, you have universal and individual needs that must be addressed in order to make the transition meaningful, productive, and positive. Having been to LPN school, you have some idea of what likely lies ahead, and returning to nursing school might be a daunting challenge.

There are times when the journey to becoming an RN seems too steep, with treacherous footing. Take a deep breath and pat yourself on the back, for you have already accomplished a great deal. You believe you can do it! Believing in yourself is the cornerstone of success. Very few people reach their goals without persistence. As you begin your journey, remember that a challenge is lost only if one ceases to try. Any effort is an accomplishment.

If asked why you decided to resume nursing education, your answers might vary from needing to improve your financial prospects to hoping to fulfill a lifelong dream. In any case, most adults seek to continue their education due to particular life circumstances, having identified needs in their lives. The desire to return to college may have been present for some time. However, not until certain conditions prevailed did resuming education become a priority.

Both internal factors, such as your personal desire or aspirations, and external factors, like the need to increase your income potential, may definitively make becoming an RN the top priority in your life. At the point at which you enrolled in nursing school, you were acting upon your **outcome priority**, the most important issue or need to be addressed at any given time within a set of conditions or circumstances. This term, which is threaded throughout this book, may be applied to virtually any situation. In the first several chapters of this book, we will be addressing your individual outcome priorities as related to making the transition back into school and from LPN to RN.

Reviewing the Past

One of the greatest strengths a person has is the realization that past experiences and accomplishments are key tools when working toward a new goal. Knowles, Holton, and Swanson (1998) describe four ways that experience influences learning. First, it develops and accentuates differences between learners. Experience is also a source for insight and motivation, but it can just as well be a barrier or a rigid mold into which new learning may have a hard time fitting. Finally, experience is the foundation upon which you define yourself. As a learner you will become part of a **cohort**, a group of people engaging in a common experience. You will gravitate toward those in your cohort whose past experiences have shaped their habits, attitudes, and other traits such that you become compatible with or complimentary to them. The experiences you and your cohort share are valuable tools in gaining understanding and perspective.

Experience can also make some learning difficult. An old concept or detail may seem clear in your mind, but it can be challenged or modified with new information. Often adults must be able to make sense of new material in the presence of previously established beliefs or knowledge. Finding critical links between what you already know and new information to integrate is a key to learning as an adult.

Experience adds layers of description to definition of the self. You may consider yourself "good" or "bad" at starting IVs based on patient reaction in the past. Such self-definition may influence your actions. You may either avoid having to start IVs or seek additional practice and instruction so that your skills can improve. Use good or bad experience as a link to new learning, and be open to the possibility of accommodating something new.

Relate each new piece of information to your daily practice. You can likely recall examples of patients or experiences in the past that will make the critical connection not only for you but also for those in your cohort group with whom you share them. Life stories are an important element in integrating new learning. These and your experiences, as well as prior learning, make up the **scheme**, or web of connections, to which all new learning must be related so that it makes sense. Work with each new concept and detail until it feels comfortable in your already well-developed scheme.

In order to move forward, you need to determine where you have been. You must closely and critically examine the path you have traveled to this point. In Exercise 1-1, briefly sketch your **experiential resume**, a concise list of your experiences and prior learning. Begin at the point of completion of your LPN program. Make a timeline, including events, accomplishments, and setbacks that stand out in your mind, detailing the surrounding circumstances and other aspects as much as possible. Looking at your experiential resume, what are some of the lessons you

---

Exercise 1-1   Experiential Resume

Secondary education completed _____ (date).

Entrance to RN school _____ (date).

learned along the way? What will you do similarly or differently as you embark upon the next leg of your journey?

Let's look at experiences more critically now. Research in adult education has determined that past experiences may either help or hinder both present and future educational endeavors (Knowles, Holton, and Swanson, 1998). Past experience may serve as a chain to which new learning may be linked, making concepts understandable within your personal context. Conversely, some experiences make learning more difficult, in that new information may contradict, and make it necessary to unlearn, previously accepted information. The process of unlearning is more difficult than initial learning.

In Exercise 1-2, separate the items you wrote in your experiential resume into either the positive impact or negative impact category. Determine the impact based on your beliefs at this time (you may always switch them later). For instance, perhaps after high school, you entered nursing school but were in an accident and had to withdraw. Maybe you were unsuccessful in your first nursing science class and dropped out. How did this likely influence subsequent decisions and actions? You might have decided that the nursing program was just not appropriate, or you might have tried to determine what needed to be done to ensure success the next time.

We leave the past for now. As we move into the present, keep your experiential resume in mind. Along the way it may be necessary to revisit the list in Exercise 1-2 to determine the roots of problem situations that may arise. Having noted both positive and negative past experiences, you have armed yourself with a portion of a key tool to success, self-awareness.

Exercise 1-2

Positive-Impact Experiences   **Negative-Impact Experiences**

Examining Where You Are Now

"The most difficult of all perspectives is to see oneself as one really is" (Wilson and Porter-O'Grady, 1999, p. 230).

Now that you have reviewed your past experiences and accomplishments, it is time to examine your current personal and professional status. To grow beyond the status quo, you must be fully able to assess who you are, your motivations, and the conditions, environment, or role that you currently occupy. How would you describe your personal self? The personal realm includes the areas of your life before and after work and those that relate to your private goals rather than company goals. What are your roles, your traits? What can be said about you professionally? That is, regarding the business in which you earn your living, how would you describe your roles and traits? In Exercise 1-3, define who you are by completing the phrases.

Now that you have defined who you are, what do you want to change? What motivates you to return to nursing school, to spend the next few years preparing yourself to become an RN?

Too many times LPNs resuming their nursing education have misjudged their current levels of knowledge, experience, and even their licensure when planning how they will go about successfully negotiating a professional nursing program. LPN school is nothing to sneeze at, and you

Exercise 1-3

I define my personal self as:

I define my professional self as:

have "been there, done that" and passed the NCLEX-PN examination. Your current licensure is evidence of your ability to succeed.

In Exercise 1-4, write what it currently means to you personally to practice in the role of an LPN. Then speculate how your practice will change as you take on the role of an RN.

Knowles, Holton, and Swanson (1998) apply Vroom's Expectancy Theory to explain that adults are motivated to learn when they believe that the outcome of that learning will be useful and important to themselves or others. In the struggle to continue, it can be easy to forget why the journey was begun. Understanding your individual motivation for resuming your education will be helpful to keep you on the right, albeit winding and occasionally uphill, path. In Exercise 1-5, explain your motivations or most important reasons for returning to school.

Exercise 1-4

Perception of Current LPN Role   **Perception of New RN Role**

Exercise 1-5

My outcome priorities and most important reasons prompting my return to nursing school are:

Setting Your Goals

"By taking the time to create a vision and a purpose for your life, you will approach your work with a broader, more critical, and more strategic outlook" (Wilson and Porter-O'Grady, 1999, p. 222).

A map can be helpful when planning a journey if there is understanding of where you have been and where you are now. It is time now to define where you are going. To avoid drifting in the sea of education, a destination must be clearly defined. It is not often that airplane tickets are bought for just any airport in a large region. The itinerary is more precise. Charting a course does not necessarily mean plotting the shortest distance between two points, however. Rather, the route should accommodate individual needs and desires. The key is to keep moving in a purposeful manner.

Determining the path begins with definition of both short- and long-term goals. A **short-term goal** may be something that could be attained in 6 months or less. A **long-term goal**, then, would take longer than 6 months. Being true to your inner self, the examination of personal goals occurs first.

In Exercise 1-6, write your personal goals. The personal realm encompasses everything outside of your professional life. Such goals might include getting married, having children, and moving into a new home. Write the goals first, then label them "ST" (short term) or "LT" (long term). Finally, prioritize them, placing the number 1 next to the most important or most immediate, the number 2 for the next most important, and so on.

In Exercise 1-7, using your professional goals, complete the same process as in Exercise 1-6.

Prioritizing

Now that you have determined both your personal and your professional goals, choose the number one short-term goal of each type and write the associated outcome priority. Remember, the outcome priority is the need or situation that must be addressed above all others for you to reach the goal. For example, consider what you have to do to accomplish the goal of going to the "rush-hour" show with your family on Friday. Several things must be planned from before the time you leave for work to the time the feature begins. Maybe you purchase theater tickets early in the week. Friday morning you take hamburger out of the freezer for dinner. You leave for work early enough to fill the gas tank. You complete your banking during lunch. These are all priorities that will make it possible to enjoy the Friday feature.

$Exercise$ 1-6	**Personal Goals**	
Goal	**ST or LT**	**Priority**

$Exercise$ 1-7	**Professional Goals**	
Goal	**ST or LT**	**Priority**

This is just an example for one family outing, but much the same process of prioritizing and planning can move you steadily toward your larger life goals. Wilson and Porter-O'Grady (1999) ask an important question: "Do you set daily priorities that move you forward toward your dreams?" (p. 221).

In Exercise 1-8, complete the statements.

The final exercise in plotting your course is the development of a time-line against which to gauge your progress. In Exercise 1-9, arrange your short- and long-term goals along the time continuum. Be sure to write down where you imagine yourself 5 and 10 years from now.

Change Theory

Similar to Vroom's Expectancy Theory, Empirical-Rational Change Theory suggests that adults will make a change if they can foresee the benefits

Exercise 1-8

The outcome priority related to my number one short-term personal goal is:

The outcome priority related to my number one short-term professional goal is:

Exercise 1-9

Present _____ (date)

5 years

10 years

that may result (Marquis and Huston, 2000; Tomey, 2000). Keeping this in mind, let's explore the process of change and how it will help move you toward achieving your goals. In 1951 Kurt Lewin described three phases of change as well as what he termed driving and restraining forces, pushing toward and away from change, respectively. Those descriptions still

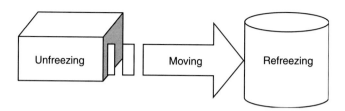

Figure 1-1 According to Change Theory, the three phases of change are unfreezing, moving, and refreezing.

apply today (Lancaster, 1999; Tomey, 2000). According to Lewin's theory, one goes through unfreezing, moving, and refreezing during the change process (Figure 1-1).

You have engaged in the process of change while working through this chapter. You have examined your needs or motivation for change as well as those forces that make change easier or more difficult. You have identified why you want to change your current life routine to include going back to college, going to clinical experiences, and the rest of what a nursing program brings. This is known as **unfreezing**. The more reasons you find that compel you to take action, here to resume your education, the more unfrozen you become. As an ice cube must be melted to water before assuming a new state, so must your current life state unfreeze for you to move toward your dreams.

You have also engaged in the second phase of change: you are **moving**, actively planning changes and taking action on them. Moving also means you are dealing with both positive and negative forces as they ebb and flow and you are making modifications to your plan as needed (Marquis and Huston, 2000).

Refreezing happens when a change becomes an integral part of who you are and what you do. This is not to imply that the change is permanent. Any change you desire must be continually renewed in order to maintain stability. Once a positive change has been integrated, a person often begins the unfreezing process again in order to begin working toward another dream or goal. Let's say that after you become an RN, you find that you especially enjoy teaching and decide that you would like to become a nursing faculty member. The new goal requires that you have an advanced or even terminal degree (MSN or earned doctorate) to achieve success.

Tomey (2000) defines eight types of change that you may experience: coercive, emulative, indoctrinizing, interactive, natural, social, technocratic, and planned. The meanings of each are embedded in the terms. The type of change in which you are currently engaged is likely the last listed, planned change. You have identified your needs, have made a plan, are implementing the plan, and will experience the integration of the change into your life as a part of this planned process.

Summary

You have completed the initial processes necessary to launch yourself in the right direction as you begin your journey. The outcome priority theme was introduced and applied to exploration of your past, present, and future self. Research in adult education has determined that past experience can both help and hinder the assimilation of new learning. Becoming aware of the positive and negative impacts of prior learning experiences prepares the learner to deal with the results of those experiences.

After thoroughly examining the past, you addressed the current definitions of personal self as well as professional self. Understanding your current positions and perceptions leaves no doubt as to the starting point for the journey and may even provide insight into potential pitfalls along the way. Finally, after assessing both the past and the present, you explored the future. You established short- and long-term goals to clearly delineate the path to your final destination. You developed a timeline against which you can gauge individual milestones along the way. To clarify the process in which you are engaged, Change Theory was introduced and applied.

Critical Thinking Questions

1. Name an RN whom you admire. What characteristics help you define him or her as an expert nurse? How would you envision your practice as an expert nurse?

2. You are attempting to balance your job, family, and work, and you are not satisfied with your grades in school.

    a. How would you describe your problem?

    b. What is your outcome priority?

    c. What measures could you take to help with the balance and meet the goal of getting better grades?

3. How is your practice legally differentiated from that of an RN in your state?

References

Knowles MS, Holton EF III, Swanson RA: *The adult learner: the definitive classic in adult education and human resource development*, ed 5, Houston, 1998, Gulf Publishing.

Lancaster J: *Nursing issues in leading and managing change*, St Louis, 1999, Mosby.

Marquis BL, Huston CJ: *Leadership roles and management functions in nursing: theory and application*, ed 3, Philadelphia, 2000, Lippincott Williams & Wilkins.

Tomey AM: *Guide to nursing management and leadership*, ed 6, St Louis, 2000, Mosby.

Wilson CK, Porter-O'Grady T: *Leading the revolution in healthcare: advancing systems, igniting performance*, ed 2, Gaithersburg, Md, 1999, Aspen.

Chapter 2

Identifying Individual Tools

Key Terms

learning styles
self-awareness
self-directedness

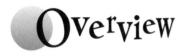verview

In this chapter you will identify your individual learning tools. In doing so, you will examine your gifts and barriers, your learning style, and your personality traits and learn how they may affect your study.

Gifts and Barriers

Many people are uncomfortable with the idea of listing their individual gifts or strengths and barriers or weaknesses. Etiquette has taught many to be modestly self-deprecating about positive attributes so as not to seem arrogant or pompous. We may also try to ignore characteristics within us that are less positive. Understanding and addressing your gifts and barriers have a twofold effect. Being aware of the traits that make you unique will both keep you from repeating mistakes and give you the ability to internally support yourself, providing the best opportunity for success.

In Exercise 2-1, list in as much detail as you wish (the more, the better) as many of your gifts and barriers as you can identify. **Self-awareness**, being conscious of and understanding yourself, is your ongoing self-portrait. It is not a measurement of what others may think of you or your performance but what you understand about yourself. This exercise will heighten your sense of yourself. Studying the self-portrait can be a very healthy experience if you are then motivated to support the strengths and

Exercise 2-1

Gifts	Barriers

work to lessen or remove the weaknesses you've identified. You may or may not choose to share such insights.

Once you have several items listed, you can prioritize them, which is necessary to keep you from becoming overwhelmed and to focus your energy where it can make the most difference. Prioritize your list items by numbering them, placing a number 1 next to what you consider your greatest gift and another 1 by your most troublesome barrier. Give 2s to your next best and next worst traits. Go down both lists, numbering each item.

Develop a statement regarding the outcome priority for both the number one gift and the number one barrier. Write the statements in Exercise 2-2. Here the outcome priority is related to the first or most important gift or barrier issue to be dealt with. For example, if you wrote "good listener" as your greatest gift, an outcome priority might be, "Apply listening skills at each class session." Similarly, if "procrastination" is your greatest barrier, then an outcome priority might be, "Seek guidance from an advisor regarding techniques and behaviors to help stop procrastinating."

Self-awareness is essential but will not give its full benefit unless you take action to correct or minimize your weaknesses and capitalize upon or maximize your gifts. Make a plan of action, a self-care plan, to specify just

Exercise 2-2

The outcome priority related to my greatest gift is:

The outcome priority related to my most troublesome barrier is:

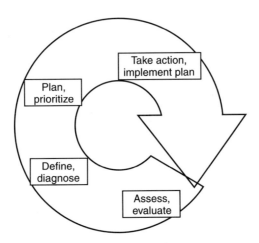

Figure 2-1   Action plan.

how to go about addressing the outcome priorities you have established. When writing the plan of action, be as specific as possible. Include target dates or time periods for reassessment. Reevaluate your plan of action periodically to determine whether changes are in order.

Note your plan's similarities to how you plan the care that you deliver to patients. Patients are assessed for needs that require intervention as well as for strengths that require support. Patients are periodically reassessed, and interventions are continued, discontinued, or modified to meet their changing health status. This process may be visualized as a succession of phases that are circular and in motion (Figure 2-1).

In Exercise 2-3, write a plan of action to support the outcome priorities for the gifts and barriers you determined earlier. An example is provided.

Return to your self-care plan from time to time, at least at each target date, to assess your progress with each outcome priority. When you revisit your self-care plan, ask yourself the following questions: "Am I making progress toward the outcomes I've established?" If not: "What can I do differently?" "Are my target dates realistic?" "Do I need more help?" If you are consistently mastering your specified outcome: "Is it time to focus on a new area?"

Writing about your experiences along the way will help. Keeping a journal is a great way to reflect upon what you learn about yourself.

Exercise 2-3

Outcome Priority (OP)	Interventions to Correct or in Support of OP	Target Date for Reassessment
Decrease procrastination behaviors.	1. Make list of all assignments.	1. End of first week of class.
	2. Prioritize list items according to due dates and difficulty.	2. Every 2 weeks thereafter.
	3. Assign work dates and time needed, place on calendar.	

Use your journal to evaluate your progress and to examine the questions that arise.

Now that you have determined gifts and barriers that influence your personal and professional identities and performance, point out other characteristics you possess that influence abilities and behaviors.

Learning Style

Many instruments are designed to help individuals better understand **learning styles**, the manners in which they prefer to learn. Many studies have attempted to correlate learning styles and the methods of teaching and studying that best suit each style category. In general, although it remains inconclusive how predictive most instruments and inventories are, they are still considered excellent tools for gaining personal insight.

Kolb (1984) developed a Theory of Experiential Learning as a cycle composed of four phases: concrete experience (CE), reflective observation (RO), abstract conceptualization (AC), and active experimentation (AE). The cycle theoretically begins with an experience, which the learner reflectively observes and conceptualizes. This leads to participating in an experiment or experience, which then begins the cycle anew. Based on this theory, Kolb developed the Learning Styles Inventory to determine individual learning style preferences. Following the responses to a 12-item questionnaire, the learner is placed into one of four categories, each having unique characteristics and preferences related to the four phases of the learning cycle. Kolb believes that as a learner matures, the preferred style becomes more of an integration of the traits of all four categories, not only the initially dominant one, such that the learner effectively moves between all of the styles as needed.

Numerous studies have applied Kolb's Learning Styles Inventory to various types of nursing students. The studies came up with different results, all of which were significant. The greatest impact, however, is likely within the individual student, as insight is gained into how to apply one's strengths. Knowing your preferred style of learning is important, but you must adapt your preferred style to the learning context.

All learning preferences are valuable, and none is considered better than the others. Preferring active experimentation, some people seem to learn best by doing, by "trying it out." Such learners may try many different solutions to a problem before settling on one. Others prefer what Kolb calls *reflective observation,* watching events or experiences without having to be directly involved. These learners are usually good listeners and prefer to bring problems to harmonious solutions. Those predisposed to abstract conceptualization are considered data organizers. These learners order and arrange information in meaningful ways and are often happier in a lecture-type format, where they will write and arrange notes to their liking. People who prefer learning through concrete experiences relish being directly involved in new experiences in a hands-on fashion. These learners are likely to solve problems as they go and are good at adapting to new situations (Kolb, 1984).

Your preferred style of learning is not restricted to the school setting. Learning takes place every day in all the places where you live your life. You likely participate in learning along the lines of each of Kolb's categories in a wide variety of activities. In Exercise 2-4, identify learning situations that would be examples of Kolb's four theoretical categories.

Exercise 2-4

Concrete Experience	Reflective Observation	Abstract Conceptualization	Active Experimentation

Personality Traits and Learning

Some researchers believe that learning styles and preferences are closely tied to personality type (Lawrence, 1993). Perhaps you have taken a survey or inventory that suggested that your personality has particular traits. The Meyers-Briggs Type Indicator (MBTI) is one such survey. Through a series of questions, the MBTI helps determine dominant personality traits: extroversion versus introversion, sensing versus intuition, thinking versus feeling, and judgment versus perception. Research states that people have and use both traits in each category but that one is displayed more than the other (Lawrence, 1993).

Most people can readily identify the difference between extroversion and introversion, which can be characterized as acting versus reflecting. Extroverts prefer to talk about things. They are seen as action-oriented, outgoing people. Introverts prefer to consider issues inwardly and privately. Extroverts prefer to have study partners and often need compelling external pressure to study. Introverts prefer to read and listen quietly, rarely asking questions or adding to the discussion.

The differences between sensing and intuition are not quite as clear. People who prefer gaining understanding about their observations through the five senses are considered sensors. Study for sensors requires relating new, abstract concepts to prior concrete knowledge. People who gain understanding about their observations abstractly and through their imagination, using their intuition, are considered intuitive. Details may escape persons who learn by intuition until they can grasp the larger concepts to which the details refer.

People who make decisions objectively are considered to prefer thinking. Thinkers need to believe that they really know the content and will study until the material makes clear sense. On the other hand, those who heavily weigh their subjective feelings while making decisions are considered to favor feeling. Those who learn through feeling will likely study with friends and spend a good amount of study time helping their friends learn the material.

A person who carries out his or her life in a manner that implies careful planning is considered to prefer judgment. Study time for this person will follow a carefully conceived plan in an orderly fashion. Conversely, a person who prefers living life spontaneously and fluidly is considered to prefer perception. Perceivers prefer to study just what interests them, when the notion strikes.

Another instrument for determining learning style is the Preferred Learning Style Index (Seidl and Sauter, 1990; Stone, 1974). This inventory categorizes students as either receptive or discovery learners. Receptive learners prefer organized, systematic delivery of information, such as in a lecture. Conversely, discovery learners prefer to arrive at information on their own through experimentation and problem solving.

A third method of determining learning style is based on Gregorc's Theory of Mediation Ability (1982). Gregorc states that "the human mind has channels through which it receives and expresses information most efficiently and effectively" (p. 5). Of these four channels, an individual will favor one over the other three. Depending on which channel is dominant, a learner will exhibit particular characteristics.

One study (Duncan, 1996) investigated differences in perception and ordering abilities based on the application of the Gregorc Style Delineator, with groups of student nurses in programs of different levels. *Perception* is the manner by which a learner takes in information. *Ordering* is the way information that has been taken in is organized and subsequently expressed or applied. A learner perceives in two ways: abstract and concrete. A learner also orders in two ways: sequentially and randomly. Completion of the Gregorc Style Delineator identifies an individual's preferred style of learning. The four possibilities are depicted in Figure 2-2 as quadrants: concrete sequential, abstract sequential, concrete random, and abstract random.

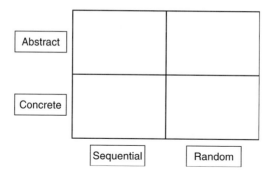

Figure 2-2   Possible quadrant results for Gregorc Style Delineator.

People who prefer the *concrete sequential* style like structure and are organized and pragmatic. They learn through memorization and repetitive drilling, such as with flash cards or verbal quizzing with a partner. *Abstract sequential* learners prefer pictures and ideas and are often considered inconsistent or highly variable in their study patterns. *Concrete random* learners prefer to study alone. They excel at distance learning, where independence is required. Computer-aided or web-based instruction will likely suit them. Concrete random learners also like to solve problems, so arranging information into case studies with conditions and questions will often help. *Abstract random* learners use their emotions and senses to grasp new information (Duncan, 1996; Gregorc, 1982).

Self-Directedness

Self-directedness has been described in numerous ways. Knowles, Holton, and Swanson (1998) identify two perspectives of self-directed learning. Persons seen as "self-teaching" (p. 135) engage themselves in the learning environment and determine the pace and methodology of study, such as in home or independent study. The other perspective is one of autonomy, or "assuming ownership of learning . . .[leading] to an internal change of consciousness in which the learner sees knowledge as contextual and freely questions what is learned" (p. 135). These two perspectives are considered independent and may be present in a learner either alone or together.

The ability to engage in self-directed learning may be considered a requirement for the nontraditional student. More programs are attempting to meet the needs of adults returning to school by increasing the amount and complexity of material provided in a learner-paced, learner-directed manner. Therefore the learner must be prepared to exercise initiative, independence, and persistence, along with the discipline and determination to meet goals and to solve problems when challenges arise. Being self-directed is not necessarily inherent but may be viewed instead as a process that requires practice, time, and experience (Merriam and Caffarella, 1999). Like most adults managing multifaceted lives, you may have come to understand that success in life outside the classroom requires behaviors similar to those identified as self-directedness. As you transition back to the role of student, assume responsibility for your educational experiences and opportunities, thus transferring those adult, self-directed behaviors into your role as a student.

Consider for a moment how you exhibit behaviors consistent with self-directedness in your daily life outside of school. List the behaviors in Exercise 2-5, then write about how you might transfer those behaviors into the learning situation.

If you understand your individual learning style as a student as well as your personality traits and preferences, then you and your instructors will be able to plan learning experiences that better suit your needs. In addition, understanding your needs as a learner, particularly related to becoming more self-directed, will empower you to take control of your learning. Capitalize on your strengths and build upon areas that require nurturing

Exercise 2-5

Behaviors	How to Transfer Behaviors into Learning Situation

for growth. Gone are the days when faculty were the carafe and students the empty vessel waiting to be filled with knowledge. Today students are responsible for their own learning, and faculty serve as guides and facilitators.

Summary

This chapter has focused on the traits you already possess: your internal gifts and barriers as well as your preferred learning style. A self-care plan was developed in order to capitalize on strengths and to correct weaknesses. In doing so, a crucial part of self-awareness was gained.

Kolb's stages of the learning cycle were explored. The four stages in the learning cycle begin with concrete experience, followed by reflective observation, abstract conceptualization, and active experimentation. This last stage leads again to a concrete experience, and thus the cycle begins anew. Understanding learning preferences further enhances opportunities and empowers you to seek experiences that speak to your preferred style of learning. Practice moving through further stages in the learning cycle, because learning is optimal when you complete all four stages.

Personality traits as identified by the MBTI were discussed, along with their implications for learning and study styles. Characteristics of self-directedness, often associated with the most successful learners, were discussed as a means to enable you to take control of the learning experience.

Critical Thinking Questions

1. The concept of professionalism is a thread throughout the history of nursing. Working in a group of at least three or four student nurses, each of you chooses a time in the history of nursing and composes a single report

comparing the significance of the past events with present nursing conditions.

2. You have identified your learning style preference. As you work in the group on question 1, note the differences in learning styles between the team members.

   a. What aspects of your learning style will be challenged?

   b. What aspects will be enhanced?

3. a. What are the potential consequences of not setting personal and professional goals?

   b. What would it look like, feel like, and seem like if you fail to reach the goals you set for yourself?

c. What measure can you implement to ensure that you will feel good about your successes even if you do not meet all your goals?

4. All reasoning begins with basic assumptions. You started this chapter with a basic assumption that your gifts and barriers will potentially help or hinder your progress toward professional development.

   a. For each of your gifts, what assumptions can you make about how it will assist you in completing your mobility program?

   b. How would you test your hypothesis that this gift will help you?

   c. What measure will you take to ensure that your barriers do not hinder your progress?

References

Duncan G: An investigation of learning styles of practical and baccalaureate nursing students, *J Nurs Educ* 35(1):40, 1996.

Gregorc AF: *An adult's guide to style,* Columbia, Conn, 1982, Gregorc Associates.

Knowles MS, Holton EF III, Swanson RA: *The adult learner: the definitive classic in adult education and human resource development,* ed 5, Houston, 1998, Gulf Publishing.

Kolb DA: *Experiential learning: experience as the source of learning and development,* Englewood Cliffs, NJ, 1984, Prentice-Hall.

Lawrence G: *People types and tiger stripes,* ed 3, Gainesville, Fla, 1993, Center for Applications of Psychological Type.

Merriam SB, Caffarella RS: *Learning in adulthood: a comprehensive guide,* ed 2, San Francisco, 1999, Jossey-Bass.

Seidl AH, Sauter D: The new non-traditional student in nursing. *J Nurs Educ* 29(1):13, 1990.

Stone HL: *Preferred learning style,* Madison, 1974, University of Wisconsin-Madison Center for Health Sciences.

Chapter 3

Personal Empowerment Skills

Key Terms

locus of control
personal empowerment
self-defeating behaviors
self-talk

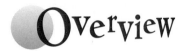verview

Empowerment means to provide a way for doing something, to set free the ability to move forward, to enable. **Personal empowerment** means giving yourself the opportunity to succeed, or enabling your own success. Being empowered can also be thought of as having a positive attitude, feeling in control of your own destiny, and believing that you are important (Nugent and Vitale, 2000).

Personal empowerment skills are behaviors that you practice to improve your ability to accomplish goals or that motivate you to engage in your education and other life activities from a position of strength and control. For the most part, personal empowerment skills are learned skills that most people do not already possess or regularly practice. They include assuming an internal locus of control, practicing positive self-talk, eliminating self-defeating behaviors, managing the work of success, and managing your health.

Assuming an Internal Locus of Control

Whether your **locus of control** is internal or external describes where you believe the power in your life resides. If you have an external locus of control, you believe that the responsibility for your actions or inaction lies outside of yourself. For example, in the case of a less-than-satisfactory grade on a test, the student may externalize the locus of control by saying, "The test was too hard" or "The instructor gave me a B." If your locus of control is internal, you take responsibility for what happens to you, for your mistakes as well as your accomplishments. Using the same example, the student with an internal locus of control might say, "I need to study harder next time to improve my grade" or "I earned a B on my paper."

In the left column of Exercise 3-1, write statements that you have made in the past that represent an external locus of control. In the right column rewrite the statement so that it reflects an internal locus of control. Discuss how this process might aid in your transition from LPN to RN.

Positive Self-Talk

People who are empowered often think good thoughts about themselves and engage in positive **self-talk**, talking to themselves kindly and with

Exercise 3-1

External Locus of Control	Internal Locus of Control

encouraging words, in a manner that would support and affirm. Consider the child faced with trying to ride a bike and repeatedly wobbling and weaving, with a near-fall here or there. A parent might relate the story of *The Little Engine That Could,* a powerful story for all ages. If you think you can and you tell yourself that you can, then you can. It feels great when someone we love, trust, or admire tells us, "Great job!" or "I am so proud of you for working so hard!"

An affirmation from yourself is also very valuable. Only you really know how much work and sacrifice went into doing something well by "giving it your all." Be as kind, understanding, forgiving, and encouraging to yourself as you would be to a fellow student, a child, or a friend who is doing the best possible. Learning is a process of forward motion but also steps back, with reflection and inner contemplation.

Tell yourself, "What I am doing is important to me and to the world. I will make a difference in my own life as well as those of others." The affirmation that is in order at this point in your education is "I can do this." When life in nursing school gets a little hectic, as it inevitably will, repeat to yourself silently or out loud, "I can do this, I can do this."

Nothing is more counterproductive than to convince yourself, "I don't get it" or "I can't do this." Negative self-talk is a damaging coping mechanism that may seem to lift the stress of a situation temporarily by claiming that what is before you is insurmountable, out of your league, or over your head. Do not allow your mind to begin to chatter such untruths. The pressure is off for a moment if you excuse yourself from facing and conquering the fear of doing what a situation requires. The pressure will only be replaced with shame and guilt or regret; however, do not allow your mind to begin to chatter such untruths.

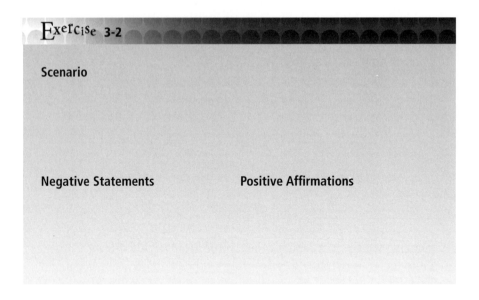

Scenario

Negative Statements   **Positive Affirmations**

You can do this. You have what it takes. You can will yourself to work through every situation. Be positive and empower yourself to succeed.

Exercise 3-2 will enable you to turn negative self-talk into positive affirmations. We have all experienced self-doubt and self-defeating behaviors. Think back to a time when you recall having said to yourself, "I cannot do this" or "I'll never get this right." Any statements about yourself that were less than positive will work here.

In Exercise 3-2, write a short but meaningful scenario. Below the scenario in the left column, list the negative phrases that likely occurred to you at that time. Then think of an affirming statement that counters each negative phrase and write it in the right column. If you are comfortable doing so, say your affirmations out loud. You may at first feel odd doing this, but this is one way to ensure that you will not experience the same negativity should the same or similar scenario arise again.

Elimination of Self-Defeating Behaviors

Another crucial skill of personal empowerment is the recognition and elimination of **self-defeating behaviors**, which put us at risk of failure. These behaviors, when routinely permitted, can lead us to fulfill the prophecies that our positive affirmations seek to counter. Chenevert (1995) describes several behaviors that directly impede our ability to succeed. These include pessimism, nit-picking, worrying, and perfectionism. Blaming is another prevalent form of negative conduct. The remedy for such self-defeating behavior, as suggested by Chenevert, may be in continually recognizing their presence in ourselves.

Pessimism

Viewing current situations and anticipating outcomes from a negative perspective, a pessimist is the type of person who views a glass of milk as half empty rather than half full. Pessimism creates the negative self-talk we seek to eliminate. The choice between pessimism and optimism in an otherwise healthy person is simply that: a choice. Choose to be optimistic.

Validating that little voice inside that says, "Be careful" or "Don't do it" is not the same as being pessimistic. Pessimism is expecting that success is not possible, no matter what the situation. Pessimism removes our power and makes us give up any control we may have over the events in our lives.

A note of caution here: chronic pessimistic behaviors and perceptions can be symptoms of a serious illness or disorder. It is best, if you find that you experience frequent pessimistic feelings, to seek the advice of your primary health care provider.

Nit-Picking

One way of rationalizing a decision that otherwise could not be supported, nit-picking is a damaging compensatory mechanism that seems to release the nit-picker from responsibility for getting the job done. A person with a nit-picking attitude seems to look for the tiniest fault. If the nit-picker chips away at small details, sooner or later the sum of all the imperfections will lead to a reason not to move forward. This may be simply a sign of uneasiness or perhaps of some undisclosed concern.

Worrying

In a similar way, worrywarts often immobilize themselves with fear. Worry wastes time and uses energy better placed into planning and proactivity. When you've done your best, listened to your internal voice of reason, and made your decisions based upon all the evidence at hand, you can stop worrying. Worrying about what might happen will change nothing, but it robs you of the energy you will need to plan for, or cope with, the outcome either way. Worrying is not action, and only action provides any hope of changing the outcome.

Perfectionism

Perhaps one of the most discreetly cloaked self-defeating behaviors of all is perfectionism. How old were you when your parent first told you, "No one's perfect"? What is it, then, that makes us believe that we must be perfect? To strive for perfection is to be perpetually unhappy, as we fall short. This is not to say that to try to improve ourselves is futile but rather that we should set goals that are humanly possible and go for them. Each time we try, we learn and are therefore closer than before. Perfection is out of the question, but continuous improvement is not.

Blaming

Shifting blame to others is one of the most destructive self-defeating behaviors. To blame is to reject the responsibility of control over outcomes, saying something goes wrong, it is someone's fault besides our own. If we are unable to accept the responsibility for our actions or inactions, we are not going to benefit from reflecting about what we could have done differently, which might have changed the outcome.

Accountability is a major creed for professional nursing. Being a nurse means accepting responsibility not only for the care you personally give but also for the care given by those under your supervision. If you are constantly looking to blame someone else, then you are not accepting responsibility for your actions and therefore not learning from them.

Managing the Work of Success

Success at home, at work, and at school is directly related to your ability to manage the work of success. Having completed a practical nursing program, you are well aware that success takes work. The four key work habits that need to be developed and maintained in order to manage your success are decision making, planning, commitment, and time management.

Decision Making

A strong decision-making ability shows that you are in control. You have settled on what you want. Stick to your decision unless you are strongly compelled to change your mind. This applies to all decisions. One decision you might make is to earn a B or better in a particular course. This is your decision. The teacher does not give you a grade; you earn it. As you read earlier, this keeps your locus of control internal.

Planning

There is no more powerful builder of self-esteem than, by the end of the day, to have accomplished all you had planned. Planning is essential to the smooth functioning of the busy life of an adult in school. Planning requires close assessment of every aspect of the task at hand and its context. What are the conditions and requirements? What instructions, parameters, or guidelines do you have?

To plan means making sure you have all the necessary resources to complete an assignment as well as have a backup plan. What are you going to do if your car breaks down on the way to the library and you lose all the time you had set aside for study that day?

Planning includes breaking down a goal into its individual parts and prioritizing them, so that you first complete the most urgent or otherwise logically first tasks. Doing well in a course involves a series of small tasks that, once summed together, equal the whole. Break your course down into separate testing periods or projects. Make each of them a separate goal, and break it down further into even smaller steps that will lead to successful completion.

We can often be immobilized by the sheer size of an entire project or task that lies ahead. Breaking a project or study session down into more manageable pieces is a strong motivator for continuing the work until it is finished. Just looking at one small part of the whole brings back your motivation. Completing one part at a time and concentrating on only that one part will eventually lead you to completion of the entire task. Before you know it, you are at the end of the semester, you've completed all the assignments, and the grade you had set out to earn is yours.

Think for a moment what it feels like after you've said goodnight to your last dinner guest, only to come to the kitchen doorway and see piles of messy dishes, a greasy stove, and an otherwise perfectly shiny floor (which you had spent 2 hours scrubbing) dribbled with drips and spills of various foods and beverages. It is all just too much to deal with. Or is it? If you separate the cleanup into its individual tasks, the job won't seem so big.

Likewise, if you have a 70-page reading assignment in order to be prepared for the next class, the time to plan is as soon as you are aware of the assignment. Examine your schedule. Determine the study time you have to devote to this assignment, then divide it up. Read and take notes on all that you had planned—and then some, if your energy level and time permit. When the next class rolls around, if you have stuck to the plan, you should be ready.

Commitment

The third habit for managing your success is commitment, or total dedication, to your plan (Watford, 1996). Commitment requires discipline. You've carefully dissected a goal into its parts, and then each part into its individual pieces. You have made the necessary assessments in order to prioritize, and you have all the necessary resources to see it through. Dedicate yourself to the plan.

Initial dedication to your plan will be wholehearted and vigorous. The challenge comes later, when you are required to maintain the plan in the face of other mounting responsibilities and waning resolve. You must have the discipline to turn away from a more attractive proposal of how to spend your evening, when you know you have a test the next morning. For example, instead of going out to a midnight movie that would interfere with a good, full night's rest, opt for a quiet evening of study and reflection that ends early, so that you can take the test the next morning fully rested and ready to do your best.

To further bolster your commitment, try to remember your original inspiration for going to nursing school. What can keep you going? Perhaps you have a picture, poem, or phrase that sums up your motivation. Keep a tangible reminder near you. Take time to reflect, take stock of your accomplishments, and praise yourself for working toward your goal.

Time Management

Unfortunately, poor time management skills can get in the way of carefully made plans by the most committed of individuals. Learning effective time management skills is crucial to success. Effective time management applied consistently can be a great asset and may be considered the box that organizes and carries all the essential study skills and other tools that you use to build your education. Planning and completing a task without your toolbox can be difficult.

Before we investigate the contents of the box, let's examine the box itself. As an LPN, you are most likely returning to school with a busy, well-established life. You no longer have the luxury of hanging out at the library every day, like you did when you first went off to school. Your home life, work life, and school life must be well orchestrated. To manage time effectively, you must learn to set and prioritize goals (Meltzer and Palau, 1997). The importance of these skills cannot be overemphasized.

ASSESSMENT Assessment is the first task to help you develop effective time management (Exercise 3-3).

SETTING GOALS AND PRIORITIZING Setting goals is the next necessary step. The goals here are different from those you developed in Chapter 2. Here we examine one semester.

In Exercise 3-4, list the activities and events you need or want to participate in this semester. This list should include things such as attending school part- or full-time, working part- or full-time, serving as den parent or room parent, volunteering, having your family over for Thanksgiving, or hosting a birthday party. Place the number 1 next to the most important thing that you must accomplish, a 2 by the second most important, and so on.

Meltzer and Palau (1997) point out that every activity cannot be the top priority. Some activities require that you change or limit others. Even during a nursing program, you must balance your goals so that you do not ignore what makes you happy.

Now that you have listed and prioritized your semester goals or activities, place them on your calendar. Most advisors agree that a key to success in college is the ritual use of this essential organizational tool. A calendar that shows days, weeks, and months is an absolute necessity. Keep it with you at all times.

Go back now to your semester goals. Note your number one priority. What do you need to do to accomplish this? For example, if working full- or part-time is your first priority, include in your schedule not only your work hours but also the time it takes to get ready, pack your lunch, and drive or catch the bus to and from work. (Remember the daily assessment

Exercise 3-3

On a separate sheet of paper, write out every activity that you do during your average day. For example, choose a Monday and complete the following:

1. List everything you do on a typical Monday, from waking up your children to brushing your teeth, making coffee, and showering. Include relaxation and personal time.

2. Next to each item, write in how much time you spend on each task. Be realistic, and do not leave anything out. At this point, you are not deciding what to change, just assessing your usual day.

3. Now add up all the time spent. The idea of time management is not to stuff 20 hours of work into 16 but to determine what needs to be done, what can be delegated to others, and what can be done differently to maximize the quality of the time you spend in each activity.

Exercise 3-4

Semester Goals   **Order of Priority**

you completed in Exercise 3-3.) Repeat this process for your second priority and on down the list.

The syllabus given out during course orientation is the key to accomplishing your school goals. Go through the syllabus and transfer class dates, times, and locations to your calendar. Block off time for travel and walking to and from the parking lot. Some other things you will want to mark on your calendar are exam dates, paper due dates, project due dates, group work sessions, study sessions, anticipated library and computer lab time, and advising and registration for next semester. Most schools expect you to study or prepare at least 2 to 3 hours for every hour you spend in class or clinical. Do not scrimp on this time. The time you spend engrossed in study will pay off when you prepare to take the NCLEX-RN.

Write on your calendar all of your personal or family responsibilities of which you are aware. These may be things such as doctor and dentist appointments; exercise class or going to the gym; taking out the garbage, doing laundry, and paying bills; family birthdays, movies, concerts, and going out to dinner; church and choir practice; doing your nails and going to the salon; and getting the car inspected and the oil changed. The personal list is endless. Refer to your average daily assessment. Can you delegate some activities on the list to another family member? While you are in school, allow others to help you. The point of time management is not to enable you to cram everything into a day but to help you choose the few most important priorities and apply quality time to those activities.

TIME WASTERS   This is the difficult part: identifying the ways you waste time. Be aware of the time you spend that is not productive. This is not to say that resting and relaxing are not productive; they are essential to keeping your body and mind functioning at their best.

In Exercise 3-5, list the time wasters that interfere with your daily productivity. After you've listed the things that steal your time, write what you believe you could do to solve each problem. For instance, if you get caught up in watching TV, talking on the telephone, surfing the Internet, visiting with friends, or reading for recreation, then set limits on the amount of time you will spend in such activities and stick to them.

Chenevert (1995) points out that procrastination may be recognized as a self-defeating behavior. Procrastination seems to accompany tasks that are difficult, are complex, or do not have immediate apparent application. Procrastination can be basically harmless, or it can be devastating. Procrastination is defined as, for any number of reasons (excuses),

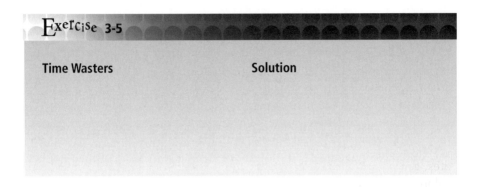

delaying or putting off an activity or responsibility until one is at or past the deadline. If you recognize that you are putting off a task, take a closer look. What about the task, specifically, causes you discomfort? Separate the whole into its parts and work with the individual pieces. If you've just been unable to find the time to go enroll in that next class, then you probably dread a specific part of the class or the enrollment procedure. Work toward resolution of the situation one issue at a time.

Time wasters are often procrastination in disguise. Not everyone procrastinates for the same reasons. Experts say that procrastination comes in many cloaks. Do you recognize any of these?

- **Paralysis by planning.**   You plan and plan to perfection but never implement. You spend so much time planning that you run out of either time or motivation to complete the task.

- **Perfection.**   Often perfection is not required, and usually it is out of reach. Some students turn in assignments late claiming that they just weren't happy with them. Work your best within a limited amount of time.

- **Boredom.**   If the task is not interesting to you, you must discipline yourself to get it done. Strive to find significance and personal purpose in every assignment.

- **Hostility.**   Perhaps you have negative feelings toward the person assigning the task, you are required to work within a group that has historically been a less-than-optimal match for you, or you are angry or upset regarding the characteristics of the assignment, such as its complexity, amount of work, or due date ("too hard, too much, too soon"). Try to remove emotion from the action needed for completing the assignment.

• **Adrenaline rush.**   Working against a deadline can provide an intense, satisfying adrenaline rush. Unfortunately, while this may serve as a positive influence for some, adrenaline junkies may find that their work does not get finished when an unforeseen last-minute complication happens. If you're likely to say, "I work better with a deadline," consider that this may mean that you need external pressure to create the urgency to force you into action. If you do your best work at the eleventh hour, then consider doing most of the work early, saving only the polishing or finishing touches for near-deadline time. In any case, the first time you miss a deadline or have to ask for an extension for an assignment that is due, you have crossed the line from a late starter–strong finisher to a full-fledged procrastinator, and behaviors must change for you to preserve both your sanity and your grade.

FYI 3-1 lists 10 ways to help you quit procrastinating.

Managing Your Health

Living a healthy life and paying attention to your personal health needs are critical to achieving self-empowerment. Students often sabotage otherwise gallant efforts by ignoring their basic needs for adequate rest, relaxation, exercise, and nutrition. As a practical nurse, you are well aware of the labor-intensive nature of the nursing profession. If you are to be able to concentrate fully on the task at hand and help those in need, you must meet your own needs first. A brain that is well nourished and well rested is a more powerful brain.

In nursing school you will learn, if you haven't already, that people who are ill or injured or lacking nutrients, hydration, rest, or shelter often feel powerless. The saying is true: "If you do not have your health, nothing else matters." In today's society, more than ever before, health equals power. At the very least, those who are trying to maintain or regain their health are considered powerful consumers and are the target of much product marketing. Think about how you feel when you are making smart choices about eating, drinking, exercise, and lifestyle in general. How do you feel when you achieve balance between work and play? You feel in control. This is how it feels to be self-empowered.

FYI 3-1   10 Ways to Quit Procrastinating

1. **Be rational.** Understand that many people can justify most any action or inaction through faulty reasoning. Examine your reasoning and separate what is true rationalization from what is false rationalization. Do this by writing down your rationale, or scheme of reasons, for believing the way you do. Beside each reason identify the source of the information. If you further identify actual fact rather than hearsay and what conditions you know to exist rather than what you or others speculate, then you are thinking carefully through your decisions.

2. **Maintain positive self-motivation.** Always speak in positives. Tell yourself, "The sooner, the better," and "I can do this."

3. **Do not predict the worst.** If you expect the worst, the worst may happen, as you paralyze yourself with fear and self-doubt.

4. **Set goals.** Be realistic and stick to the plan.

5. **Prioritize.** Begin each day by dealing with the number one priority. Remind yourself of what must be accomplished.

6. **Break it down.** Large tasks will often overwhelm you into immobility. Take the project apart and assign each part, in order of priority, to a different block of time or date.

7. **Organize your life.** Nothing wastes more time than disorganization. The time invested in getting organized will be rewarded exponentially.

8. **Commit.** Publicly committing yourself to a task or project, by sharing with a friend, relative, or classmate, often keeps you on track. You will have more trouble slacking off if you know others are expecting you to complete the job.

9. **Employ reminders.** Often we forget that we "were going to do something." Whether this was a conscious or subconscious act is not really important. What is important is that we remember. To improve your chances of remembering, put obvious notes around your house, at the office, or in your car.

10. **Celebrate.** There is nothing like positive reinforcement to keep a good thing going. Give yourself a pat on the back after every accomplishment.

Stress and Stress Reduction

One of the most disabling experiences of nursing school is a high level of stress, which seems to affect every nursing student at some point. To some, mild stress is a motivator, but to others, even mild stress on top of an already complicated life is nearly lethal.

STRESS   Sources of stress are many and varied. While research has identified common causes and manifestations of stress, every person experiences stress and the stress response differently. Commonly reported stressors for student nurses include significant others, finances, and grades (Twiname and Boyd, 1999).

Significant others experience their own stress as you progress through college. They may feel neglected or burdened when school responsibilities require you to give up time with family and friends. You in turn will feel the result of that stress. Children, spouses, and other family members and friends will vie for your attention in ways that are positive and not so positive. To help relieve the tension, be sure to block out time throughout every week just to be with your significant other, and keep it sanctified. Let nothing interfere with that time, so that each minute is quality time. Hold family meetings to discuss what it means for you and for them that you are back in college and working hard. Do the same with friends. Keep everyone up to date on your progress and let them know how they are helping to make your success possible.

Finances and work responsibilities are among the most worrisome stressors for adult students returning to school. As an adult, you have a life that is well established and, as such, already full of responsibilities that require you to manage a delicate balance between work and home, which school only complicates. Furthermore, returning to school is an expensive endeavor. Not only does it involve added costs for tuition, fees, books, and uniforms, but nursing students also find that they must cut back the number of hours normally worked to have time for classes, clinical, projects, and study. Financial assistance is available in the form of grants, scholarships, and loans; however, to receive assistance you must ask for it. You must often complete interviews and paperwork to qualify. Ask your advisor or school financial counselor about how to access the many types of financial assistance available.

Grades seem to be a major source of stress for many students. The minimum acceptable grade in nursing school is higher than that in many other programs of learning, and earning a D is just not acceptable. Many students must maintain a certain grade point average to keep a scholarship. This puts a great deal of pressure on the student. In addition, some students are not happy with anything below an A, which is just not reasonable for many. Give yourself a break. Be happy, but not complacent, when you have done everything you know how to do, have given your all, and still received a B or a C.

If you do not have command of a topic, study it until you do, even after the test. Nursing education is designed to build on prior learning, documented or not. Some people are among the world's top nurses despite grades lower than A's in nursing school, likely because they did their best when in school and continued to work at it until they fully understood what they needed to know.

STRESS REDUCTION   Just as the manifestations of stress are individual, so too are the techniques that aid in stress reduction. What works beautifully for one person may serve to add stress for another. The literature generously reports coping mechanisms and techniques to reduce stress. Holistic cognitive therapy, however, engages a process that may lead an individual to optimum stress reduction. Four steps are involved in cognitive therapy (Dossey et al, 2000):

1. *Achieve awareness.* You achieve awareness through understanding how you feel under stress. How does your body physically feel? Does your headache or your shoulder feel tight? Maybe your stomach gets queasy, or you lose your appetite. Maybe your appetite increases. Become aware of the early signs of stress and take steps to reduce or neutralize the symptoms.

2. *Identify automatic thoughts.* These are usually immediate responses made without reflection. They have formed before we even realize the entirety of a situation. They are almost always negative in nature, with hard or blaming words like *should* and *never* correlating the discomfort directly to an outside source, real or imagined. Automatic thoughts are usually distorted and irrational, with little or no basis in reality. The only way to deal with automatic thoughts is to acknowledge the possibility of their existence and to identify them as what they are.

3. *Identify cognitive distortions.* These are illogical, irrational thoughts. Look carefully at the following list of 10 cognitive distortions and

try to identify any of these in yourself during a past (or present) time of stress:

- *All-or-nothing thinking.* This includes thoughts such as, "If you cannot be the best, then you won't be anything at all," or "Anything less than perfect equals failure."

- *Overgeneralization.* This involves lumping all similar situations, events, or people into broad (usually negative) categories.

- *Mental filtering.* This is manifested by identifying one negative detail and then characterizing the whole by that one part.

- *Disqualifying the positive.* This is characterized by the inability to see positive experiences as important or by refusing to accept compliments on a job well done.

- *Jumping to conclusions.* This is identified as "mind reading" or acting or making decisions without evidence.

- *Magnification.* This involves making a problem seem worse than it actually is. The converse, failure to see the importance of what went well, is also a cognitive distortion.

- *Emotional reasoning.* Just because you believe or feel a certain way, that does not make it so. A distorted way of thinking is to confuse feelings with fact.

- *"Should" statements.* Although statements that contain the word *should* are meant to bring about action, they seldom do.

- *Labeling.* When a person, situation, or event is labeled, it is automatically characterized and burdened inappropriately with the characteristics of others within the category.

- *Personalizations.* These are manifested by placing yourself at the center of everything. If you are personalizing, you feel that everything negative that happens in your world is all because of you.

Scary, isn't it? Facing the reality behind the façade of cognitive distortions is neither easy nor without pain. Accept yourself as you are without the façade and work from there. There is no right or wrong or judgment to be passed, only an opportunity to get to know yourself so that you can empower yourself to succeed in a world that is unpredictable and imperfect.

4. *Choose coping mechanisms that work.* To come up with an appropriate response to a stressor, you must identify both the practical side of the issue, the factual information surrounding the situation, and the emotional side, how you feel about it. They will likely each need a different method for effective coping. Following is a list of mechanisms that may help you cope:

- *Distraction.* Deciding to lay aside the stress until it is necessary to deal with it is not a means to avoid the situation but to reserve the angst until such time as the situation can be dealt with directly.

- *Direct action.* There is something you can do to resolve the problem.

- *Relaxation.* Employ techniques or activities that bring about relaxation at the initial awareness of stress. This can help change your physical and psychological responses as well as the action taken either proactively or in response.

- *Reframing.* Looking at the situation from another perspective often sheds a different light on it and can alter your behavior within the moment. This may also be referred to as, "looking for the silver lining."

- *Affirmation.* A positive thought is an affirmation. As you learned previously, thinking positively can benefit the outcome. People who think they can, can!

- *Spirituality.* One very powerful means of coping is to think deeply about what feeds you spiritually. Turning to your faith may help you put life back into perspective.

- *Catharsis.* Crying and laughter are both often helpful as emotional releases.

- *Journal writing.* One safe way to bring out thoughts and feelings and work through them is on paper. Writing can be an effective means of processing stressful situations.

- *Social support.* Sharing with family members or friends is an effective means of dealing with stress for many people. Talking about stressors often leads to learning not only new ways to cope but also ways to avoid stress, where possible, by changing behavior.

- *Assertive communication.* Your ability to communicate needs and desires clearly is important for others to be able to respond appropriately.

- *Empathy.* Being able to put yourself in the place of another helps you understand them.

- *Acceptance.* Forgiveness and letting go of those things that are beyond your control helps you maintain balance when you are unable to alter or avoid the situation.

This list is not an all-inclusive grouping of techniques but a place to begin the process of cognitive therapy, a most personal voyage toward self-empowerment.

Summary

Becoming empowered is an active process. Empowerment cannot be bestowed upon you (although you may feel motivated by others); rather, you achieve it. Five basic skills are required for enabling your success:

1. Assuming an internal locus of control
2. Engaging in positive self-talk
3. Eliminating self-defeating behaviors
4. Managing the work of success
5. Managing your health

The moment you begin to engage in self-empowering behavior, you will feel the surge.

Critical Thinking Questions

1. Your patient needs an IV started for antibiotic therapy. During report you learn that the patient is a difficult IV start and that the RN leaving the shift, one of the most skilled IV starters, tried to start the IV two times without success. You walk into the room and introduce yourself and are introduced to the patient's son and daughter, a nurse and physician. Write a brief but honest narration as to how you feel about this situation.

a. What will be the consequences if you do not have positive self-talk going into this situation?

b. From the patient's point of view, what are the main concerns related to the IV?

c. What could you do to put a positive and supportive spin on this event?

2. You have clinical on Tuesdays and Wednesdays, with clinical paperwork due Thursday morning at the beginning of class. This paperwork generally takes you 2 hours to complete. Although you have been keeping up with the daily class assignments, you would like to schedule some study time. This week you have a unit exam scheduled on Thursday at 0900. Your study group wants to meet Wednesday evening before the unit exam.

a. What decisions must you make?

b. What will your action plan need to look like for you to complete the work as well as study for the exam and meet with your study group?

      c. What will be your top priority and lowest priority? List potential conse-
quences to your selections (remember, *consequence* is a neutral term, so
list both positive and negative consequences to your prioritized items).

3. Reframe the following statements or concepts to be positive:
    a. The glass is half-empty.

    b. This door is closed to me.

    c. The cardiovascular unit is too hard to understand.

    d. The clinical instructor is always picking on me.

    e. I cannot get to class on time; I am always running behind.

    f. I could not understand what she was talking about, and then when she
asked me the question, I looked like such a fool.

    g. I would like to believe I passed the exam, but what's the use?

    h. I don't know what I did to make her angry, but she'd better get
over it.

    i. What is the matter with me? I stayed up all night preparing to complete
this clinical assignment, and then I get it all wrong.

References

Chenevert M: *Mosby's tour guide to nursing school: a student's road survival kit*, ed 3, St Louis, 1995, Mosby.

Dossey BM et al: *Holistic nursing: a handbook for practice*, ed 3, Gaithersburg, Md., 2000, Aspen.

Meltzer M, Palau SM: *Learning strategies in nursing: reading, studying and test-taking*, ed 2, Philadelphia, 1997, WB Saunders.

Nugent PM, Vitale BA: *Test success: test-taking strategies for beginning nursing students*, ed 3, Philadelphia, 2000, FA Davis.

Twiname BG, Boyd SM: *Student nurse handbook: difficult concepts made easy*, Stamford, Conn, 1999, Appleton & Lange.

Watford L: *How to study and manage your time effectively when working on the Distance Learning Program*, CUNY Distance Learning Program, New York, 1996, City University of New York.

Section 2

Becoming a Successful Student

Chapter 4

Classroom Study Habits That Work

Key Terms

major details
minor details
multiple-choice
  questions
SQRRR
structured-response
  questions

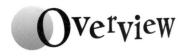verview

Chapter 3 discusses two crucial actions that support self-empowerment: affirmation and the elimination of self-defeating behaviors. Self-empowerment yields fruitful results when paired with a few helpful study habits. Success in college is directly related to your success at developing and maintaining basic study skills.

Even adults need to practice classroom behaviors that promote learning, and they don't necessarily come naturally. This chapter defines skills and tools to help you get the job done.

General Classroom Behavior

You'll be better off sitting near the front of the classroom and away from distractions. Resist the urge to talk, unless you are working with a group or engaged in discussion with the class or instructor. If you are tired, bored, or prone to daydreaming, look over previous notes until you can focus on what is going on in the classroom. Copy down each key word and diagram the instructor puts before you. If it is important enough for a professor to write down, take that as a clue and include it in your notes.

Effective Listening

Listening is not the same as hearing. It is a conscious activity that requires a number of skills.

Before Class

Before going to class, prepare for what you will be hearing not only by reading the assigned material but by reviewing your notes from the previous class.

During Class

Listen and watch for cues that will indicate when the instructor is about to say something he or she does not want the class to miss. Maintain a positive attitude. Even if the teacher makes statements that you disagree with, do not spend the next several minutes thinking of your rebuttal; rather, jot down a word or two and continue to listen. When the time is appropriate, add your comments to the class discussion. Do not remain passive in class. Gaining meaning from new information requires that you interact with it. Ask questions, and actively work with the information while it is new, until you are clear. Make it a practice not to leave class with unanswered questions or if you are confused regarding topics or assignments. Maintain your concentration. Think about what is being said. If you are not attentive, your memory will dump the information before you can hook into it. Allow flexibility. Most teachers provide an outline or agenda in some form for each class meeting. However, if the class is allowed to depart from the plan, do not panic. Stay with the discussion. If you truly begin to lose your train of thought, then ask a question for clarification. This may help both you and the teacher get back on topic.

Immediately After Class

At the end of the session, spend a few minutes reviewing the notes you just took. Add additional clarifying comments. Try to find the answers to any questions that come to mind.

Effective Note Taking

Oddly enough, some students ask, "Do we need to take notes on this?" The answer to that is always a resounding "Absolutely, yes!" Never miss an opportunity to record what you are learning. Simply hearing a lecture or participating in an experiment or project is not enough for anyone. To fully understand what is being said, you need to be able to review it and reflect upon all that has transpired. Most human short-term memories will dump any material that has not been processed within minutes of the event.

Before Class

Read the outline and prepare yourself for what you will hear. You can do this the same way you prepare for listening. Complete your reading assignment before class. Review prior notes and be ready to listen when class begins. Make sure you have plenty of paper and at least two pens or pencils with you in the classroom. Have them out and ready. You do not want to miss anything or bother classmates while you root in your bag for spares.

During Class

Do not try to record a verbatim transcript of the class. Instead, paraphrase what is being said. Write key words and phrases, especially unfamiliar terms, titles, and concepts. Use acronyms and symbols or your own version of abbreviations to increase speed. (Caution: use only abbreviations with which you are familiar; otherwise, you may have a page of gibberish at the conclusion of the lecture.) Write legibly. Use underlining, highlighting, or stars to indicate areas that the presenter signaled as most important. Include examples, pictures, diagrams, and formulas. FYI 4-1 lists common verbal signals often used by instructors to indicate important information.

FYI 4-1   Common Verbal Signals

Most instructors signal, either consciously or subconsciously, what they believe to be most important. Common verbal signals include the following:

- Numbering items ("First, . . . Second, . . .")
- Pointing out the main idea ("Most important . . .")
- Highlighting concepts ("Remember that . . . The basic concept is . . .")
- Giving examples ("For instance, . . .")
- Changing direction ("On the other side of the coin, . . .")
- Repetition
- Referring to text
- Changing tone of voice
- Using qualifying words ("Always," "Never," "Rarely," "Often")

After Class

As soon as possible after class, review and expand your notes. You will likely need to add words and phrases and fill in other gaps to give your notes detail.

- Write down any points that you may remember from class that you do not have in your notes. Make connections to content that was covered in prior classes.

- Compare notes with a classmate.

- Develop your own test questions related to the material for later review.

Effective Reading

One of the most important steps you will take toward a successful college experience is improvement of your reading skills. Nursing programs have always been, and will always likely be, text oriented and reading intensive. Among the most important keys to effective reading are maintaining your concentration through active reading, identifying main ideas, relating details to a main idea, highlighting appropriately, and improving reading speed.

Maintaining Concentration

Choose an environment for your reading that minimizes distraction. Make it clear to family and friends that for your planned reading session, you are not to be interrupted unless there is an emergency. Turn the phone ringer off and let the answering machine intercept your calls.

As in other study situations, do not get too comfortable. Textbooks are known to be dry and less than engaging; you must therefore make the effort to stay engaged in what you are reading (Meltzer and Palau, 1997). One strategy to help you stay focused is to continuously search for the presence of the main idea and related major and minor details (Meltzer and Palau, 1997). The active search keeps you involved and attentive. If you find that you are falling asleep or your mind is wandering in spite of your best attempts to remain engaged, consider that it may be time for a short break. (Caution: Limit your breaks to 10 or 15 minutes to avoid procrastination.)

Identifying Main Ideas

Isolating the main ideas of topics is paramount to comprehension. To help you find a main idea, ask yourself questions such as "What is the most important issue or point about this topic?" Most authors signal their main ideas with headings, bold type, or italics. Watch for these cues as you skim the pages before reading in depth. Once you have placed a mental flag or asterisk next to the main idea, look for details that support this idea (Meltzer and Palau, 1997).

Relating Details to a Main Idea

As you build your mental picture or outline, add the supporting details as bullet points under the related main idea. (Note: If creating a mental picture is difficult for you, write it down as you go along.) Details help you more fully understand the main idea by providing facts, descriptors, or parameters (Meltzer and Palau, 1997).

Not all details are equally important. Textbooks are often very detailed, much of the time providing so much detail that it becomes difficult to differentiate major from minor details (Meltzer and Palau, 1997). **Major details** are clearly associated with the main ideas and are often considered of primary importance. They should be the focus of note-taking and highlighting. **Minor details** are usually present in support of the major details or only peripherally related to the main idea.

Highlighting Appropriately

Underlining or highlighting your text can be a beneficial tool if you use it appropriately and judiciously. Highlighting is meant to aid in later review. The following are basic guidelines for highlighting written material:

- Read the entire section at least once before you highlight. If you try to underline the first time you read the section, you will often end up underlining entire passages, which will not benefit you when you review.

- Try to create your own sentences by highlighting only certain key words or phrases. Leave out unnecessary words. You may need to write a few of your own words in the margin to make the highlighted words and phrases flow smoothly.

- Try to highlight no more than 20% of the material. (For example, if a section has 50 lines of text, highlight no more than 10.)

- Use different ways of highlighting—circles, underlines, asterisks, stars, arrows—to indicate differences in the material.

- Regularly review the material you have highlighted. If you are unable to answer study questions with something you have highlighted, go back and reread the entire passage to look for missed points.

Improving Reading Speed

Evidence relates reading speed to comprehension: the faster you read, the more you understand what you are reading. The same skills may be associated with both increased comprehension and the ability to read material quickly. You can improve reading effectiveness and efficiency by identifying and reducing factors that inhibit reading (FYI 4-2) and by promoting the good habits that enhance reading rate and comprehension (FYI 4-3).

Alter your reading rate according to the type of material. Reading for enjoyment is different from reading for analysis. Although you may read

FYI 4-2   Reading Inhibitory Factors

- Having to read aloud or word by word

- Unfamiliar vocabulary or jargon

- Difficulty making smooth line changes with eyes

- Reading the same material over and over, also called *regression*

- Lack of engagement with or attention to what is being read

- Lack of experience with reading the amount or type of text you are expected to read

- Trying to remember everything

- Forcing reading acceleration rather than improving reading habits

FYI 4-3   Improving Reading Conditions and Habits

- Make a visit to the optometrist or ophthalmologist. Many times a slow reading rate and poor comprehension are related to visual defects.

- Try not to sound out words during reading. First prepare yourself by going over key terms. Practice saying them aloud until you are comfortable with both their pronunciation and their spelling. Then, as you encounter them in your reading, you will be less likely to stumble and regress (have to reread).

- Stay engaged and focused as you read. Allowing your mind to wander encourages regression and a slower pace, which sets you up for more distractions and regression, and an hour later you've read one paragraph.

- Practice using a broader eye span: look at more than one word at a time. Text is meant to be read as long, streaming sentences and passages. Focusing on one word at a time (or reading word by word) is distracting and inhibits your ability to focus on the idea being presented.

novels extremely quickly yet with thorough understanding, you will likely find it necessary to decrease your speed for detailed or technical information. Do not become frustrated at needing to reread to gain complete understanding of nursing and other scientific texts. Frequent review is a necessary part of the discipline for both beginners and experts.

Skimming and Scanning

Among reading tools that are especially effective for reading nursing and scientific texts are skimming and scanning. Nursing texts are generally packed with data and details, and students crawl through the underbrush searching for main points and for what is a "must-know" versus a "nice-to-know." By practicing skimming and scanning before your in-depth reading, your retention of major concepts, ideas, and details will improve (Meltzer and Palau, 1997).

To effectively read a chapter or passage, you must first skim to locate its main ideas or the main concept. This provides the skeleton that you will flesh out with necessary information as you read for depth later.

Scanning locates unfamiliar or key terms and phrases. It also calls your attention to concepts that are new to you. Scan for definitions, formulas, and pictures that represent or support main ideas.

Improving Your Study Skills

The following is a five-step method for studying that has been used for many years: survey, question, read, recite, review (**SQRRR**). If applied consistently, the SQRRR formula will help you thoroughly study your material.

Step 1: Survey

To survey means to skim the book. Read the headings and subheadings along with the lead sentences that go with each. Read each chapter summary and introduction. Write down any unfamiliar terms as you survey.

Step 2: Question

Make questions out of the headings and subheadings of each chapter and write them down. Instead of writing "Steps in the Nursing Process," write, "What are the steps of the nursing process?" Write a question for each main idea in the chapter. Use any study guides the teacher provides.

Now answer your questions the best you can without returning to the book. Try to reinforce your understanding of any new or unfamiliar terms as you consider the answers to the questions.

Step 3: Read

Read the first section of the book, searching for the answer to the first question you wrote. You may underline a key word here or there. After you have read the entire section, write out what you have found to be the answer to the question. Use your own words. If some terms cause you to stumble, change them, as long as you understand the meaning.

Step 4: Recite

Without looking at the book or your notes, try to say aloud in your own words your explanation or answer. If you are unable to do this just yet, look over the section, your question, and your written answer again.

Repeat steps 3 and 4 with each section of the chapter. Continue until you complete the assigned reading.

Step 5: Review

Once you have completed the entire lesson this way, review daily by reciting aloud the major points of each section. The three stages of review or study are early review, intermediate review, and final review.

Early review is the most efficient and productive form of review. Before you go to class or read new material, do the following:

- Refresh in your mind prior material.

- Say out loud the major concepts of what you already know.

- Engage in early review immediately after class or reading the new material, because review makes the most sense when it is associated with what you already know or have very recently learned. Forgetting happens most quickly immediately after learning. Planning time to engage in early review directly after class is essential.

- Rework your notes. This does not mean to copy—that won't help. Merge the notes you took in class with notes you jotted down during study.

- Organize what you learned by drawing arrows, pictures, or graphs, adding any memory cues that come to mind.

- Associate what you have just learned with what you already know. Speak out loud and link new concepts with prior concepts. In nursing the curriculum builds, so you should be able to write out how what you've just learned relates to what you already knew.

Taking place after early review is completed, intermediate review focuses on understanding the material. Intermediate review is especially important when you have several weeks before an exam.

Final review takes place in the days immediately before an exam. This is not cramming; final review is not the time to try to catch up on unlearned material. Rather, recite aloud to yourself or a study partner everything you recall regarding the entire semester's material. Space your review sessions. Three 20-minute sessions are more beneficial than one 60-minute session.

More Study Strategies

The following are some short, straight-to-the-point tactics and strategies for getting the most out of your studying:

- For every hour of class, spend 2 to 3 hours studying.

- Start your study sessions with the most difficult or boring subjects. We all gravitate toward what we like or what is comfortable and familiar, but you must force yourself to spend quality time working toward understanding the tough stuff. You can't get away with saying, "I just don't get it." You must get it, and the only way to do that is through practice and repetition.

- Do not study for hours on end without breaks or pull all-nighters. Short but frequent study sessions are much more productive. Give yourself and your brain a chance to relax.

- Get up early. Many people are most productive before 9 AM. Your focus will be sharper and your mind clearer. (This assumes, of course, that you went to bed at a decent time.)

- Don't waste your waiting time. Take your notes along in the car and wherever you go. Instead of daydreaming or reading last year's celebrity magazine at the dentist's office, whip out your notes and review. You'll be surprised how important these short, impromptu study times will become.

- Tape the class and listen to it in the car, while you exercise, or while shopping.

- Employ what you've learned to avoid distractions. Claim your right to a conducive study environment, whether at school or at home.

- Study in a group, if possible. Not everyone is a social learner, but we all have different talents for understanding the text and applying experiences. As such, group study is great for processing new information. Studying in groups not only gives the advantage of relating information and concepts in a fun, nonthreatening environment, but it also keeps you from procrastinating because you know your group is counting on you. However, you should avoid the pitfall of being distracted by social conversation while studying in a group setting.

Finding the Balance

Nursing students often become completely immersed in the rigors and requirements of nursing school. Soon you may find that you feel as though your entire life and those of your family members revolve around your class and clinical schedule. You may also find that you feel that all you ever do is work.

Recognize that balance is important to your success. Not only do you need to devote time, energy, and attention to your work and study, but you must also give quality time to your other relationships and interests. To keep your family members and friends as well as yourself from burning out, plan time for nurturing. You are at the beginning of a new start in life, or at least in for a dramatic change. You want to be able to enjoy it. Reward yourself and your supporters on a regular basis. Maintain your health through a good diet and regular physical activity. Maintain your spirituality. Enjoy the process and experience of growth and becoming.

Test-Taking Skills

Specific knowledge about types of test questions and how to approach them can be of benefit to the test taker. The three types of questions you may encounter in didactic testing are structured-response, restricted-response, and essay questions.

Structured-Response Questions

In **structured-response questions**, the correct answers are supplied along with incorrect responses, and the test taker must make selections from those provided. Types of structured response questions are multiple choice, true-false, and matching.

MULTIPLE-CHOICE **Multiple-choice questions** are common in testing throughout nursing education and are predominant on the national licensing exam. A multiple-choice question is made up of the stem and the options, each of which is discussed in detail here.

Question Stem. The stem is the part of the item that asks the question or presents the problem and any conditions that apply. It may be in the form of a complete or incomplete sentence. Polarity, whether it is positive or negative in nature, is also an important characteristic of the stem. A positively formatted question asks about something that is true. Positive stems are used to determine whether the test taker understands information that is factual and is able to discern related information or actions accordingly. For example, the stem in the following test question is formatted in a positive manner:

You are about to begin a sterile dressing change with your patient. The first three actions you take, in order, are:

a. Wash your hands, gather your equipment, don your sterile gloves.
b. Gather your equipment, open sterile packages, wash your hands.
c. Explain procedure to the patient, wash your hands, gather your equipment.
d. Explain the procedure to the patient, gather equipment, wash your hands.

Conversely, a negatively formatted question asks about something that is false. To identify stems with negative polarity, look for words such as "not," "never," "except," "least," or "contraindicated." Negative indicator words will not always stand out, so it is a good practice to underline these and other negative words so as not to miss them (if writing on the test is allowed). The item writer usually employs a negatively formatted question when the test taker must demonstrate the ability to discern exceptions, errors, and inaccurate or inappropriate information or actions. For example, stem in the following test question is formatted in a negative manner:

In the elderly, all of the following conditions predispose the patient to urinary tract infection except:

a. Incomplete emptying of bladder.
b. Decreased renal perfusion.
c. Thinning of epidermis.
d. Relaxation of pelvic floor muscles.

The stem may also identify a priority, which you can find by looking for words such as "best" and "first." The options for this type of question stem may all appear to be appropriate, but the top priority is the key. You will be required to determine which is most appropriate or which comes first. The earlier example of a question written in a positive manner is also an example of a question asking you to decide which comes first, second, and third in a series. Because the stem of a multiple-choice question must provide all the data required to answer the question, you likely will find hints that may lead you to the correct answer.

While reading the stem be sure to understand who the object of the question is. It is not always going to be the patient or the nurse. One key to success with the multiple-choice question is to read the stem carefully and clearly understand what is being asked.

Question Options.   The options are the possible answers in a multiple-choice question. Each test item has one best or correct option. The item also has multiple incorrect options, known as *distractors* because they are created with the intent to distract the test taker from the correct answer. This increases the chance that the test taker choosing the best option is likely not a coincidence.

Many characteristics about the options might help point out the correct choices. Be wary of options that make wide, sweeping statements. Rarely can we say in nursing that one size fits all. Instead, look for options with detailed or narrow scopes. Another hint is to look for separate options that contradict each other. Either one is correct and the other a distractor, or they are both incorrect. If the options all seem reasonable, then reread the stem. You likely will have missed a key word in the stem that points to polarity or priority. At all times while considering the options, remember the basic premises upon which nursing stands: the patient is always the top priority. This may help you when your study or other test-taking techniques have fallen short.

TRUE-FALSE   In the true-false type of question, the test taker must determine whether the statement is completely true or completely false. Numerous variations on the true-false format exist; however, regardless of the variation, true-false leaves no room for shades of truth or falsity. The correct or best response should be clearly either one or the other. Read the statement slowly and carefully before choosing.

MATCHING   Most often in a matching question, the author arranges the information in the form of two lists or columns. Examine both lists carefully to determine the general relationship between the items in each list. Then, consistently using the same column as your starting point, look for matches you recognize to be absolutely correct. As you make matches, cross them off the list. Once you have made the "guaranteed" matches, then work with those you are unsure of.

Restricted-Response Questions

Several forms of restricted-response questions exist. Two familiar types are completion, or fill-in-the-blank, and short-answer questions. The item writer employs these types to test understanding of facts, definitions, formulas, and straightforward concepts. The learner is expected to provide the key words, phrases, or sentences that complete a statement or to provide the answer to the question. The instructor will look for specific information that is considered correct. However, when you are in doubt as to a specific answer, the best rule of thumb is to write more rather than less in the hope that you will supply the desired information. The following example is in the form of a short-answer question:

Laboratory data that may indicate the presence of an infection include an elevated _____, an elevated _____, and the presence of _____ in the cultures.

Essay Questions

The third major type of question you will likely encounter is the essay question, which is most often reserved as a tool for evaluating the student's ability to analyze, synthesize, and solve problems with very complex concepts and related conditions and information. To succeed with essay questions, you must be able to articulate in writing what you know. This requires not only that you have a clear grasp of the material but that you have honed your organizational and writing skills such that you are able to communicate your response effectively.

When responding to an essay question, organize your thoughts with an outline that is in the same order as the question. Then write all relevant information you have pertaining to each area of your outline. An essay answer requires more than simply a list of unrelated thoughts, however. Your answer must flow and then end in a clear summary that restates your conclusions. If you recognize that writing is not one of your strengths, you will do yourself a favor by asking your instructor or advisor for assistance. Some colleges have writing labs with faculty members or other tutors who can help you improve your writing ability. The nursing profession requires that we be able to express ourselves clearly through writing with everything from patient charting and care planning to papers and articles for school courses and publication.

Universal Advice for Optimal Test Performance

Several strategies and behaviors before and during a test may improve your performance. *Preparedness* is the main word to remember. Prepare your body, mind, and spirit by following your usual routine in the days before the test. Get plenty of rest and a well-balanced diet. All-nighters rarely produce acceptable results. By the time you begin the exam, your brain will be so exhausted and your body so far out of sync that your performance will suffer. The night before, pack everything you will need during the exam so your morning departure is not delayed as you run through the house searching for your calculator or favorite ink pen.

On the day of the exam, help reduce your anxiety by getting to the class on time. Give yourself plenty of time to relax before you begin. Do not get pulled into last-minute study sessions with classmates, but rather meditate or collect your thoughts.

Once the exam begins, read all the instructions and scan the entire test. Note how much time you have to spend on each question. Answer every question, even if you are having to make educated guesses. Leaving a question blank offers no possibility of getting it right. Some instructors offer partial credit, particularly on short-answer or essay questions, so give it your best shot.

Before turning in your test, check your answers. Reread each question and make sure you have marked the option or written the answer you intended. Marking wrong answers by mistake can be easy, particularly on tests where you must fill in bubbles or ovals to indicate your answers. Check them carefully. Make sure that any erasures are complete and that all writing is legible. Once you have turned in your test, tell yourself that you have done your best, and let go of the anxiety. Soon you will start studying for the next one.

Summary

Part of empowering yourself to be successful in school is to practice good habits that lead to effective class and study time. In the classroom you should maintain an active, positive perspective. Effective listening and note-taking skills are essential. You can improve study time through practiced and effective reading. You must be able to maintain concentration, identify the main ideas, and relate details to the main ideas. You can improve reading and understanding through greater speed and appropriate highlighting. Reading ability and comprehension are also affected by conditions and habits. A specific systematic approach to studying is suggested as one effective tool. One of the most important ways to facilitate learning is in maintaining the delicate balance between work, school, home, and play. Practicing specific test-taking techniques and behaviors can significantly improve your testing performance.

Critical Thinking Questions

1. A bird and a cat are sitting on a fence post. The bird is a good distance away from the cat, aware of its perilous perch. The bird looks at the cat and says, "Do you always need to act like a cat?" The cat replies "What do you mean?"

    The bird further ponders its position and chooses its words carefully: "By nature, you want to eat me. This fact is true. But you were raised in a caring and loving household, where you were fed and kept warm. As I sit here on this fence, I believe that if I let you get too near me, you would take my life, because that is who you are."

    The cat looks at the bird and in a shrewd manner says, "You're right. I have had a good life, have not had to hunt for my food, and am provided for in a quite luxurious way. But you are also wrong. I have no reason or inclination to want you dead or to eat you. To prove it, come sit next to me. I will not harm a feather on your back."

    The bird wisely flies away. As it is leaving it says, "You are a cat, I am a bird, and I will live to see you tomorrow because I know the difference."

    a. Explain the main idea of this story.

b. What assumptions can be made from this story?

c. Explain the point of view of the cat, then that of the bird. Is there another point of view? Explain.

d. Explain the line of reasoning used by the bird, then that by the cat.

2. For the following scenario (in quote marks), formulate at least eight questions that will help you understand what has happened. Look at your questions and see whether you have made any assumptions.

"You walk into your patient's room and find the patient on the floor."

This scenario is incomplete, which you will find to be true for most nursing situations where you will need to make decisions. Each decision you make will require you to gather as many of the facts as you can, and to gather facts, you must be able to ask questions.

3. You wake up the morning of clinical to find that your 3-year-old child has a fever of 102.3° F and is complaining of a "hurt in my throat."

   a. What is your top priority?

   b. What conflicts are you facing?

   c. What steps must you take to meet the requirements of clinical?

   Having skipped your class, your clinical instructor calls and notifies you that you have no clinical absences left and will need to consider your options.

   d. What questions do you need clarified?

   e. Write out a script of how you will discuss your options and needs. Identify assertive and nonassertive statements you have written.

f. Write a plan to meet the objectives of clinical in an alternate way.

References

Meltzer M, Palau SM: *Learning strategies in nursing: reading, studying and test-taking*, ed 2, Philadelphia, 1997, WB Saunders.

Chapter 5

Arranging and Accessing Support for Your Professional Move

Key Terms

Internet
learning resource centers
mentor

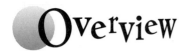verview

In the previous chapter you examined the organizational and study skills necessary to optimize your learning experience. This chapter focuses on the external support and resources—personal, professional, monetary, and academic—that are available to bolster your professional move.

Personal Support

Adults often resume education as a result of a life-changing experience. In many cases, the returning student is already under stress related to the trigger that sent him or her back to school. You should arrange for the personal support necessary to manage the addition of school responsibilities to your already busy life. Embarking upon an endeavor such as nursing school requires commitment on the part of your family and friends, as well as yourself. The student who rallies supporters prior to starting school is wise, but any time is a good time to discuss the implications with the people in your life.

Nursing education is demanding and often inflexible, producing stress not only for you but also for those supporting or depending on you. As you move back into the role of student, your friends and family members will also experience transition. Your significant other will fill new and expanded roles during the semesters to come. Although it may not be easy for you to relinquish control or accept help with certain aspects of your life, consider that it may also take special sacrifices on the part of others to take over some of those responsibilities. In moving through this period of transition, keep several key points in mind:

- Assess your personal support system, listing each person and group and the specific types of support they are able to give.

- Honestly assess your limitations. Your family members and friends may not realize the extent of your new needs, so be open in your communication with them. Before school begins, look critically at how you will spend each day. Write this down and share it with supporters so they can get a clear picture of your needs.

- Be clear in communicating your needs, and remember that others have needs too.

- Create a schedule so that your supporters can adjust their routines to accommodate their extra responsibilities. This also helps clarify the limitations of your supporters.

- Plan ahead to allow your supporters to plan ahead. If your schedule changes such that your supporters' schedules must also change, give them as much advance notice as possible.

- You and your supporters will experience much less stress if your schedule gives you a little breathing room. If you might not make it home from clinical in time to meet the school bus, then plan for that so you don't have to call someone at the last minute.

- Keep your supporters updated on your progress. They will take more pride in your success and feel as though the sacrifices they are making are worth the effort if they can hear about your experiences.

- Your supporters will be critical to your success, but you may also take them for granted when the going gets tough. Let them know now that you appreciate their efforts and express how valuable they are.

Professional Support

As an LPN you have likely established a professional network and support system. You must not only inform your colleagues but involve them as well. By this time, if you are working, you have no doubt arranged with your supervisor for the time you need off for school. Aside from scheduling, registered nurses with whom you work can be valuable support resources through your studies. They've been through it and can often empathize, offer words of wisdom, and bring a particular concept all together for you. The nurses with whom you work will probably appreciate the opportunities to help you and to refresh their own memories.

In addition to the informal network of professional resources, you will be well served to seek a relationship with a **mentor**, or a helper. A mentor can be anyone, but we usually choose someone whom we perceive to be knowledgeable and experienced within the area of our lives for which we are seeking guidance. A mentor may play one or more of the following roles (Shea, 1997):

- Listener

- Adviser

- Comforter

- Director

- Door opener (to opportunity)

- Supporter

- Friend

- Inquisitor

- Critic

In short, your mentor will help you change, adapt, and above all, grow.

Just as mentors have different roles, different types of mentoring relationships exist, depending on the duration and formality of the relationship (FYI 5-1).

A *highly structured, short-term* mentoring relationship usually is formal and has specific goals, such as during an employee orientation period. A *highly structured, long-term* mentoring relationship is often in place when an employee or apprentice is being groomed to take over the mentor's position. This may be arranged by a corporation as a part of officer succession planning (Shea, 1997). An *informal, short-term* mentoring relationship is spontaneous and may be a one-time occurrence or as needed. Often such a situation happens in response to a triggering event or a change that

FYI 5-1 Mentoring Relationships

Formality	Duration	
	Short	**Long**
Casual	Informal, short-term	Informal, long-term
Rigid	Highly structured, short-term	Highly structured, long-term

needs to take place. An *informal, long-term* mentoring relationship is also called *friendship mentoring.* The mentor meets a variety of needs over a long period of time.

Chances are, you have had one, if not most, of these four different kinds of mentoring relationships. Mentoring is an essential tool not only for successful transition back to school but also as you move from the role of LPN to the role of registered nurse. Seek out a mentor with whom you are comfortable and are able to share. Not every person you admire will make a good mentor. Mentoring requires specific attitudes and skill sets that are conducive to supporting a new professional. Should you feel that your mentor is not supporting you adequately, find a new mentor.

Monetary Support

When returning to nursing school, you receive many new challenges, not the least of which is addressed in the question, "How do I pay for this?" When you were advised regarding which classes to take, you were probably also advised that working full-time, or even part-time, would make your educational experience more of a challenge. Your advisor might have even said, "There's no way you can work full-time and do well in this program." A few days later you received a bill in the mail for an amount that made your skin crawl.

Have no fear. Help is near. Accessing monetary support for nursing school is not as difficult as it may appear to be at first. Most professional schools, colleges, and universities have financial aid counselors to assist you in garnering the support you need. Keep the following points in mind as you look for sources of funding:

- Make appointments with your school's financial aid officer or counselors. Helping you find the means to finance your education is in the school's best interest, and they will do all they can to ensure your success.

- Fill out all forms completely and submit them on time. Most financial aid counselors will tell you that the entire process begins with completing the paperwork. Make sure you have your current year's tax forms and all other vital financial records on hand and in order.

- Apply for every scholarship and grant for which you qualify. Books filled with scholarship information are available at most university and public libraries.

- Familiarize yourself with what is required to maintain each scholarship or grant. Many grants and scholarships are contingent upon grade point averages or class rankings.

- Be diligent in your search for alternative funding strategies. Many schools offer assistance exploring a variety of financial aid options, which may include the following:

  - Federal Pell Grant

  - Federal Supplemental Educational Opportunity Grant (FSEOG)

  - Federal Work Study Program

  - Federal Stafford Loan Program

  - Federal Plus Loan

  - Veterans' benefits

  - ROTC Tuition Living Assistance

  - Scholarships from both nursing and non-nursing charitable organizations

Academic Support

Your school wants you to succeed. Your success equals the school's success. Most schools therefore have on campus or on a website a place you can visit for access to academic resources. Not only will you find information on study strategies, time management, test-taking skills, stress reduction, and the like (similar to what Chapter 4 provides), but you can also find professionals trained to help you achieve success in school.

Learning Resource Centers

About 54 million Americans have identified disabilities (National Council on Disability, 1999). This number would probably rise sharply if all students were tested. However, testing for learning disabilities in adults is strictly a voluntary process, and adults are more likely to ignore such difficulties, saying, "That's just the way I am."

If you have experienced difficulty in school in the past in spite of your best efforts, you owe it to yourself to be tested for learning disabilities. Many **learning resource centers** or counseling centers offer testing. If testing uncovers a disability, you will receive assistance to accommodate your needs. Counselors are often available to give academic and personal assistance. In the case of no disability, you will be offered opportunities for remediation of skills such as reading, writing, and mathematics.

Faculty

Faculty members are often the best sources of supporting your progress in specific courses. They have a responsibility to help you gain the knowledge, experience, and skills necessary to complete the NCLEX exam successfully and subsequently to practice in a competent manner. They will expect you to meet their high standards, but they will also help and guide you as you stretch and climb to reach those standards. Get to know your teachers and let them get to know you. You have an investment in common.

Libraries

The library at or available to your school should become as familiar as your own living room. The library is packed with everything from textbooks and journals to computers, learning stations, and often Internet access. Most schools give a tour of introduction to the library. Get oriented, get familiar, and make it your business to be able to do the following:

- Complete a search for a topic using CINAHL (Cumulative Index of Nursing and Allied Health Literature) or MEDLINE.

- Find articles using the citations and abstracts given in CINAHL or MEDLINE.

- Locate a book or bound article shelved in your library.

- Request interlibrary loans for books or journal articles not found in your library.

- Access and view material stored on microfiche.

Most importantly, get to know your librarians. They are gold mines of information and provide precious links between you and the literature you need to supplement and update your knowledge base.

Textbooks

Textbooks are required. Purchase your textbooks early, and begin reading as soon as possible. Try not to purchase a used textbook with a lot of high-lighting or underlining. Don't be in a hurry to sell your textbooks, for they will come in handy for review down the road. However, textbooks are usually not your best sources for cutting-edge information.

Journals

Journals are the sources for up-to-the-moment research. The two kinds of journals are opinion, or popular, and research. When you use journal articles to prepare nursing school papers and studies, choose articles with hefty reference lists. This is usually a decent indicator that the authors have done their homework. Both kinds of journals have a place in nursing; just be aware of whether you are reading opinions or results of research.

Computers

Working with computers is a necessity in most schools, where they are often housed in labs and libraries. You will do yourself a favor by taking courses that prepare you for the computer applications in your school. Many programs are now requiring formal courses in computer science. The NCLEX-RN exam is computerized, as are most review courses. You will have to face that computer when you're done with school and off to the workplace, so you'll be better off extinguishing any computer and media anxieties you may be harboring.

Internet

The **Internet** is burgeoning with information that can help you during college. Thousands of websites are dedicated to nursing and are main-tained by individuals, corporations, and other organizations. Learning to surf the web efficiently is becoming a required skill for students.

An associated skill is determining which websites are reliable and which are not. Some information on the web is only opinion, although it may appear in a factual format. Be aware of the difference and rely on sites that are from reputable organizations known to be leaders in the field.

Many colleges now offer, as part of their nursing programs, not only web-enhanced courses, which use the Internet and e-mail to some extent, but also entirely web-based instructor-led or student-paced courses. Even completely web-based undergraduate nursing programs are available as an alternative education-delivery mode. A word of caution before you enroll in web-based courses, though: Make sure you are planning on spending as much or more time as you would in an instructor-led classroom course. Taking a course over the web does not equal less work. It often requires even more discipline and self-directedness in learning.

Summary

Many external resources are available to help you attain your goal of successfully completing a registered nursing program. This chapter has discussed many of the personal, professional, monetary, and academic support systems available to you. You are responsible for accessing these resources and gaining the benefits they have to offer.

Critical Thinking Questions

1. You are having difficulties with your nursing school assignments; you feel that the reading material is overwhelming you with the amount of information you must learn. You have tried a number of techniques, including flash cards and outlining chapters, but you believe that you just can't figure out what is important to know and what is not important. The last exam you studied for proved to be frustrating because you believed that what you learned was not on the exam, even though you found the information in the reading after the exam was complete. You decide to utilize the learning resource center to get help, but you feel this is admitting that you are not "smart enough" to figure it out for yourself.

a. What can you do to put a positive spin on seeking help?

b. What are the potential consequences of seeking and of not seeking help?

2. Office hours for your instructor are posted, but you have conflicts with the posted times and would like to set an appointment for another time. You heard that another student went to the instructor's office without an appointment and was seen.

   a. Would you consider doing the same thing?

   b. What may be the consequences of just showing up without an appointment?

   c. What would be the best time to approach the faculty member for an appointment?

d. When is the best time to set up the appointment?

e. Does the department have a central appointment desk and secretary?

3. Decide whether each topic listed below is broad enough for writing a 10-page report, a 20-page report, or a 30-page report. For each one you believe to be too broad, rewrite the topic, narrowing its focus to fit a 10-page report. Complete a literature search on one of the topics, gathering information from as many sources as possible, such as found on the Internet, at the library, and in the bookstore.

   a. Financial aid assistance for adults returning to work

   b. Support groups for individuals returning to school

   c. Ways to gain support for professional development

   d. All the responsibilities of adults returning to school

References

National Council on Disability: FYI 106#9. Washington, DC, 1999, Author. Available at www.ncd.gov.

Shea GF: *Mentoring: a practical guide,* Menlo Park, Cal, 1997, Crisp.

Chapter 6

Basic Math Review: Preparing for Medication Calculations

Key Terms

denominator
divisor
drip factor
improper fraction
lowest common
    denominator
numerator
proportion
ratio
reducing fractions

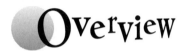Overview

This chapter reintroduces some basic math functions encountered on a daily basis by most practicing nurses (FYI 6-1). Fractions, ratios, and proportions are examined and applied. Equivalent conversions between the metric, household, and apothecary systems of measurement are crucial concepts to be practiced. You will learn about the formula method of calculating medication dosages. Basic intravenous therapy calculations are also presented.

Remembering the Basics

Fractions

A fraction is a common way of showing a number divided into equal portions. It is made up of two parts, the numerator and the denominator, separated by a line.

The **numerator** is the top number when a fraction's dividing line is horizontal, the left number when the line is a slash. It represents how many portions of the whole are represented. The **denominator**, the bottom or right number, gives the total number of equal portions. In other

---

FYI 6-1   Importance of Accurate Medication Calculation

Both the LPN and the RN must calculate medication in a consistently accurate manner. Differences in the roles are specific where certain medications and intravenous therapies are concerned. Each nurse must know his or her practice limitations, which are set minimally according to the practice acts of each state and in some cases more stringently from facility to facility. Be sure to read and thoroughly understand the policies and procedures related to medication administration in your facility.

words, the denominator represents how many parts the whole has been divided into. Thinking of the denominator in this way helps you understand the fraction line's function. The fraction line indicates that the top number is divided by the bottom number.

Example: Figure 6-1 shows a whole circle and a circle divided into four sections. In the circle on the right, $\frac{3}{4}$ of the circle is shaded. The numerator, 3, represents 3 portions of the whole. The denominator, 4, indicates that the circle has 4 equal portions.

REDUCING FRACTIONS   You may recall the term *reduce* associated with fractions. **Reducing fractions** means finding the smallest numbers that can represent the numerator and denominator without changing the fraction's value. You must be able to divide some number into both the numerator and the denominator.

Example: Reduce $\frac{12}{16}$

$\frac{12}{16}$ can be reduced by dividing both the numerator (12) and denominator (16) by 4. $12 \div 4 = 3$, and $16 \div 4 = 4$, so $\frac{12}{16}$ is reduced to $\frac{3}{4}$.

IMPROPER FRACTIONS AND MIXED NUMBERS   An **improper fraction** has a numerator greater than the denominator. When you reduce an improper fraction, the result will be either a whole number or a whole number plus a fraction, which is termed a *mixed fraction,* or *mixed number.*

You often have to change mixed numbers to improper fractions and improper fractions to mixed numbers when solving equations. To change an improper fraction to a mixed number, then vice versa, follow the steps in the examples.

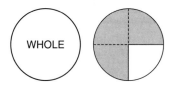

Figure 6-1   A circle as a whole *(left)* and a circle divided into four equal sections *(right).*

Example: Change the improper fraction $\frac{10}{3}$ to a mixed number.

Divide the denominator into the numerator: $10 \div 3 = 3$ remainder 1.
The mixed number is the whole number, 3, plus the remainder, 1, over
   the denominator, 3.
The answer is $3\frac{1}{3}$.

Example: Change the mixed number $3\frac{1}{3}$ into an improper fraction.

Multiply the denominator by the whole number: $3 \times 3 = 9$.
Add the result to the numerator of the fraction: $9 + 1 = 10$.
Put this result over the denominator of the fraction: $\frac{10}{3}$.

LOWEST COMMON DENOMINATOR   Another function you must
master to add and subtract fractions is finding the **lowest common
denominator**, which is the lowest number into which all denominators in
the problem can be evenly divided. Keep in mind that the lowest
common denominator may be one of the denominators presented in the
problem. Be careful not to overlook that.

Example: Find the lowest common denominator of $\frac{3}{4}$ and $\frac{2}{3}$.

   Are either of these denominators evenly divisible by the other? No.
What is the lowest number that is evenly divisible by both denominators?
To find it quickly, multiply the two denominators: $4 \times 3 = 12$. The lowest
common denominator is 12. (Note, however, that the result of multiplying
to find a common denominator can sometimes be reduced. For example,
the lowest common denominator of $\frac{1}{4}$ and $\frac{1}{6}$ is not 24 but 12.) Change
each fraction to a fraction of the same value with the lowest common
denominator, 12.

Divide the lowest common denominator, 12, by the denominator in the
   first fraction, $\frac{3}{4}$: $12 \div 4 = 3$.
Multiply the result by the numerator of the fraction you are converting:
   $3 \times 3 = 9$.
Put the result over the lowest common denominator: $\frac{9}{12}$, which is a
   fraction with equal value to the original fraction, $\frac{3}{4}$.

   Following the same conversion procedure with the second fraction, $\frac{2}{3}$,
the resulting equivalent fraction with the lowest common denominator is $\frac{8}{12}$.
   Using a combination of the preceding methods, you are ready to
apply such mathematic functions as adding, subtracting, multiplying, and

dividing to fractions. Remember that to add and subtract fractions, you must find the lowest common denominator and convert all fractions within the equation to their equivalents.

ADDING FRACTIONS   To add fractions, whether simple (a fraction with no associated whole number) or mixed, first find the lowest common denominator and convert the fractions to equivalents. Add the numerators and put the result over the lowest common denominator. Always remember to reduce your answer fraction to its lowest terms.

Example: Solve $\dfrac{1}{4} + \dfrac{2}{3}$

Multiplying the denominators, you find that the lowest common denominator is 12. Thus,

$$\frac{1}{4} = \frac{3}{12} \text{ and } \frac{2}{3} = \frac{8}{12}$$

$$\frac{3}{12} + \frac{8}{12} = \frac{11}{12}$$

This answer is already reduced. It cannot be converted to an equivalent fraction with lower numbers.

SUBTRACTING FRACTIONS   To subtract a fraction, you must also have the lowest common denominator for all the fractions in the equation. Subtract the second numerator from the first and place the result over the lowest common denominator. Then reduce, if applicable.

Example: Subtract $\frac{1}{3}$ from $1\frac{1}{2}$. That is, solve $1\frac{1}{2} - \frac{1}{3}$.

Change the mixed number into an improper fraction: $1\frac{1}{2} = \frac{3}{2}$.

Apply the lowest common denominator, 6:

$$\frac{3}{2} = \frac{9}{6} \text{ and } \frac{1}{3} = \frac{2}{6}$$

$$\frac{9}{6} - \frac{2}{6} = \frac{7}{6}$$

If the final result is an improper fraction, like $\frac{7}{6}$, for clarity you may want to convert back to a mixed number:

$$\frac{7}{6} = 1\frac{1}{6}$$

Note: Always use common sense by looking at your derived answer to determine whether it "seems" right. For instance, since we converted the final answer back to a mixed number, it is easy to see that the final answer, $1\frac{1}{6}$, is slightly less than the initial larger figure, $1\frac{1}{2}$. While this technique does not prove that your answer is correct, it can point out a blatant mistake.

MULTIPLYING FRACTIONS   Multiplying fractions does not require conversion to the lowest common denominator. Follow the steps in the example.

Example: Solve $\frac{3}{4} \times \frac{1}{2}$

Multiply the numerators: $3 \times 1 = 3$
Multiply the denominators: $4 \times 2 = 8$
Put the numerators' result over the denominators': $\frac{3}{8}$
Reduce if possible, but $\frac{3}{8}$ is already in its lowest terms.

Canceling is a process that can make multiplying fractions easier. Canceling reduces each pair of opposite numerator and denominator to lowest terms.

Example: Solve $\frac{3}{16} \times \frac{4}{6}$

Instead of just multiplying the numerators and the denominators ($\frac{3}{16} \times \frac{4}{6} = \frac{12}{96}$), first reduce to the lowest common divisor (the number by which another number is divided) of one numerator and the other denominator, then that of the other pair. The lowest common divisor for 3 and 6 is 3, and the lowest common divisor for 16 and 4 is 4. The equation now looks like this: $\frac{1}{4} \times \frac{1}{2}$, which equals $\frac{1}{8}$.

DIVIDING FRACTIONS   The trick to dividing fractions correctly is inverting the **divisor**, or the second fraction in the equation. The phrase to remember is "invert and multiply." Follow the steps in the example.

Example: Solve $\dfrac{3}{4} \div \dfrac{1}{2}$

Invert the divisor, $\dfrac{1}{2} : \dfrac{2}{1}$

Multiply the first fraction: $\dfrac{3}{4} \times \dfrac{2}{1} = \dfrac{6}{4}$

Reduce: $\dfrac{6}{4} \times \dfrac{3}{2} = 1\dfrac{1}{2}$

Ratio and Proportion

A **ratio** is another way to represent a fraction. The ratio 1:10 is the same as $\frac{1}{10}$, which is the same as $1 \div 10$. This ratio is read, "1 to 10."

A **proportion** is an expression with two ratios separated by two colons, as with $3:6::4:8$. The proportion is read, "3 is to 6 as 4 is to 8." In the preceding example, the 3 and the 8 are the *extremes,* and the 6 and the 4 are the *means.* This is important to know in order to solve proportion problems. When one of the numbers in a proportion is unknown, it is represented with an x. Thus we solve for x. Follow the steps in the example.

Example: Solve for x in the following: $4:12::6:x$

Multiply the means: $12 \times 6 = 72$
Multiply the extremes: $4 \times x = 4x$
Put the number with the x on the left and the other on the right for the new equation, separated by an equals (=) sign: $4x = 72$.
Divide both sides of the equation by the number associated with x, which is also called isolating the x:

$$\frac{4x}{4} = \frac{72}{4} = 18$$

The result is $x = 18$, so replace the x in the proportion with its derived value. The proportion now reads, "4 is to 12 as 6 is to 18." Each side of the proportion is a ratio equivalent to $\frac{1}{3}$.

Conversions of Units of Measurement

One of the most problematic areas for nursing students is converting amounts between the different systems of measurement that are widely used in health care. On any given day the average nurse must convert doses from metric and apothecary units to household units to help patients understand their medication dosages. The nurse must also calculate amounts of medicine to give when they are ordered according to a different measurement system from how they are supplied.

METRIC SYSTEM   The *metric system* is the most common system of measurement encountered by nurses. Metric amounts are expressed with decimals rather than fractions. Orders of 10 are associated with prefixes appended to unit names. FYI 6-2 provides a list of metric measures of weight, volume, and length.

You must memorize the information provided in FYI 6-2. There is no alternative or shortcut. Using the ratio and proportion method learned earlier, follow the steps in the example below to figure the conversion.

Example: Solve 2 g = _____ mg.

Write the equivalent of grams to milligrams: 1 g : 1000 mg.
Put the known from the equation in ratio to the unknown: 2 g : x mg.
Write the two ratios as a proportion: 1 g : 1000 mg :: 2 g : x mg.
Multiply extremes and means: $1x$ = 2000 mg, or x = 2000 mg.

HOUSEHOLD MEASUREMENTS   *Household measurements* are seen not only in acute care settings but more frequently in the home and home care settings. To communicate appropriate measurements to patients, who most likely use and understand household measurements, you must be able to convert metric to household and back. FYI 6-3 provides a table of conversion of metric measures to household measures.

As with conversions between metrics, you must memorize the information contained in FYI 6-3. Use what you have learned about ratio and proportion to follow the steps in the example below.

Example: Solve $1\frac{1}{2}$ tsp = _____ ml.

FYI 6-2   Metric Measures of Weight, Volume, and Length

Weight

1,000,000 micrograms (mcg) = 1 gram (g)
1000 micrograms (mcg) = 1 milligram (mg)
1000 milligrams (mg) = 1 gram (g)
1000 grams (g) = 1 kilogram (kg)

Volume

1000 milliliters (ml) = 1 liter (L)
1000 liters (L) = 1 kiloliter (kl)
1 cubic centimeter (cc) = 1 milliliter (ml)*

Metric Measure of Length

1 meter (m) = 1000 mm = 100 cm
1 centimeter (cm) = 10 mm = 0.01 m
1 millimeter (mm) = 0.1 cm = 0.001 m

---

*The abbreviations *cc* and *ml* should not be used interchangeably. Milliliters (ml) should be applied only to liquids, whereas cubic centimeters (cc) should be applied only to solids and gases.

Place what we know to be the equivalent for tsp and ml in the proportion: 1 tsp : 5 ml.

Combine the known and the unknown from the equation: 1 tsp : 5 ml :: $1\frac{1}{2}$ tsp : x ml.

Multiply extremes and means: $1x = 5 \times 1\frac{1}{2}$. (Remember how to multiply mixed numbers? Look back in the text to give yourself a hint.)

$$\frac{5}{1} \times \frac{3}{2} = \frac{15}{2} = 7\frac{1}{2} = 7.5$$

Therefore x ml = 7.5 ml.

FYI 6-3   Conversion of Metric Measures to Household Measures

Metric Measure	Household Measure
1 milliliter (ml)	15 drops (gtt)
5 milliliters (ml)	1 teaspoon (tsp)
15 milliliters (ml)	1 tablespoon (Tbsp)
180 milliliters (ml)	1 cup (c)
240 milliliters (ml)	1 glass
1 kilogram (kg), or 1000 grams (g)	2.2 pounds (lb)
2.5 cm	1 inch

Formula Method of Dosage Calculation

While some RNs and LPNs are taught to use ratio and proportion (as just presented) or to solve dosage equations, others are taught the formula method or another technique. Depending on the area in which you choose to work, you may need to use multiple methods to calculate medication dosages accurately. If you have previously learned a method that consistently gives correct answers, then stick with it.

However, if you have not previously tried using the formula method, you may find the following explanation helpful and wish to try this method out. There are many ways to explain how to use the formula method accurately. You might have encountered the formula method in one of the following forms:

$$\frac{D}{A} \times Q = x, \text{ or } \frac{D}{H} \times V = x$$

The first of these formulas is read, "The desired (or ordered) *dose* over the medication *available* times the *quantity* of the available dose equals the amount to give, or x." The second is read, "The desired *dose* over the medication on *h*and times the *v*olume of the available dose equals x."

Apply what you have learned about ratio and proportion, along with the formula method, to follow the steps in the example.

Example: The physician orders amoxicillin 250 mg. You have 125 mg capsules. How much do you give? (While this example may seem simplistic, it is a good opportunity to determine whether you are able to exercise the formulas.)

Place the ordered dose over what is available, or on hand: $\frac{250}{125}$.
Multiply that by the volume of the on hand (in other words, on hand we have 125 mg per one capsule): $\frac{250}{125} \times 1$, so $250 \div 125 = 2$. $x = 2$, so you would give two capsules.

Many times it will be necessary to convert from apothecary to metric or between other measurement systems. Conversion needs to be done before using the formula. The units of the ordered dose and the on-hand or available dose must match before you try to calculate the dose; otherwise, you will make a critical mistake.

This method of dosage calculation will work with basic computations as long as you complete the appropriate conversions first. As you find it necessary to calculate dosages and IV rates in more advanced or specialty settings, such as intensive care or pediatrics, you will need to learn calculation methods specific to those areas. For more practice in calculating basic medication dosages, refer to Appendix A in the back of this book for more exercises.

Intravenous Calculations

When IV therapy is ordered, the nurse must check to make sure all the necessary information is contained in the order, including the kind of fluid and the amount of fluid over a given amount of time. The RN is responsible for ensuring that IV fluid therapy is initiated and maintained in a safe and accurate manner. IV therapy may be delivered using either gravity, with a controller device, or a pump, which exerts pressure and does not require gravity for infusion.

To initiate IV therapy, after checking the order, you must know the **drip factor**, or established number of drops that the IV solution set (tubing) will deliver per 1 ml of fluid. This drip factor is usually found on the manufacturer's packaging. The two general types of solution sets are macrodrip and microdrip. The macrodrip delivers 10, 15, or 20 drops per ml (gtt/ml), and the microdrip delivers 60 gtt/ml of fluid.

You must also be able to calculate the following three quantities: milliliters per hour (ml/h), milliliters per minute (ml/min), and drops per minute (gtt/min). **Do not forget to include the unit with each number when solving formulas.** You will later be able to eliminate, or cross out, units as you reduce the terms of the equation.

Milliliters per hour is calculated using this formula:

$$\frac{\text{total volume to be infused (ml)}}{\text{total amount of time (h)}} = \text{ml per hour (ml/h)}$$

Milliliters per minute is calculated using this formula:

$$\frac{\text{(ml/h)}}{60 \text{ min/h}} = \frac{\text{ml}}{\text{min}}$$

Drops per minute is calculated using this formula:

$$\frac{\text{ml}}{\text{min}} \times \text{drip factor} = \frac{\text{gtt}}{\text{min}}$$

Example: Mrs. Grace is to receive 500 ml of NS over 10 hours per IV. The tubing has a 10 gtt/ml drip factor.

1. 1000 ml ÷ 10 h = 100 ml/h
2. 100 ml/h ÷ 60 min/h = 1.66 ml/min
3. 1.66 ml/min x 10 gtt/ml = 16.6, rounded up to 17 gtt/min

Here is another quick formula that incorporates all three preceding steps:

$$\frac{\text{total volume} \times \text{drip factor}}{\text{total minutes}}$$

Example: The physician order for Mr. John reads, "1 L RL over 8 hours IV. The drip factor is 15 gtt/ml."

Here you must first convert 1 L to 1000 ml and 8 hours to 480 minutes. Then apply the formula:

$$\frac{1000 \text{ ml} \times 15 \text{ gtt/min}}{480 \text{ min}} = \frac{15{,}000}{480}$$

$$= 31.25 \text{ gtt/min, which rounds to } 31 \text{ gtt/min}$$

These formulas can be used with main infusions as well as piggybacks or secondary sets. Accuracy is critical. Once you have made your calculation, think about it. Does it make sense? If you are unsure, ask another nurse to check your math.

Summary

This chapter reintroduced the basics of math associated with calculating medication dosages and basic IV therapy infusion rates. RNs encounter multiple scenarios each day that require the ability to convert from one system of measurement to another quickly and accurately. Understanding these applications of fractions and ratio and proportion are essential to safe practice. Medication errors occur in alarming numbers and in most cases are completely preventable. These mathematic skills must be perfected by every practicing nurse. Take it upon yourself to assess your math ability and act upon your findings.

Critical Thinking Questions

1. A patient receives a medication at 1 g IVPB every 12 hours (q12h). The medication comes in a unit dose of 1 g in 250 ml and, according to the

manufacturer's recommendation, should be administered over $1\frac{1}{2}$ hours. The medication pumps are all in use, and you must use a primary tubing with a 15 gtt/ml factor. At what rate (in gtt/min) must the IV run?

a. What interventions would you institute if your patient were at risk for pulmonary edema?

b. The patient has one IV line, and the IVPB is incompatible with the continuous IV medication, which cannot be stopped for the duration of the IVPB. What needs to be done? What if the patient was a difficult IV start?

2. You have a 3-year-old pediatric patient who weighs 35 pounds. You are to give a medication 30 mg/kg/24 hours in divided doses q8h. The unit dose medication comes in a 75 mg/ml of liquid. How many ml would you need to give your patient per dose?

a. What would you do if your patient had a 22-gauge IV needle in the hand?

b. The patient complains that the IV hurts. What is your intervention?

3. Your patient is to receive morphine sulfate 4 mg IVP for breakthrough pain q2h PRN. The patient is on a continuous morphine drip at 4 mg/hr from a PICC line, with a morphine sulfate concentration of 50 mg in 50 ml. Over an 8-hour shift the patient receives 3 PRN doses. What is the total mg of morphine sulfate the patient received for the shift?

   a. The patient has not had a bowel movement in the past 3 days. What interventions must be made?

   b. The doctor has indicated that the patient is to have MS Content PO after the patient's first bowel movement. What is the equivalent dose of the MS Content PO to the IV dose the patient has been receiving?

References

Ogden SJ: *Radcliff and Ogden's calculation of drug dosages: an interactive workbook*, ed 6, St Louis, 1999, Mosby.

Section 3

Understanding the Difference Between LPN and RN

Chapter 7

Differentiating the Roles

Key Terms

adaptation theory
associate's degree
bachelor's degree
developmental theories
diploma
doctoral degree
master's degree
nursing theory
role theory
scope of practice
systems theory

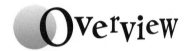
Overview

A crucial concept to explore and fully understand is the difference between the licensed practical, or vocational, nurse and the registered nurse. This chapter points out differences in educational preparation, licensure, and practice, including discussion of both the National Council of Licensure and Examinations (NCLEX) examinations and theory utilization.

Although this chapter makes conceptual distinctions between the different types of nursing, the process of adjusting one's thinking and behavior requires more than conceptual understanding. Making the transition from LPN to RN requires continuous, conscious practice and evaluation of your values and beliefs.

Educational Preparation

Because you are already a licensed practical nurse, you are well aware of the schooling required for you to be eligible to take the NCLEX–Practical Nurse (NCLEX-PN) examination. You likely received your LPN education in a hospital, high school, vocational or technical school, or junior or community college. Although the programs have variations, the minimum standard for each program is set by the individual state nursing board, whose goal is to produce graduates with a common base of knowledge and experience that will prepare them to practice as safe and competent beginners.

Only one registered nurse designation exists, with a common nationwide definition. The American Nurses Association (ANA) has defined nursing as "the diagnosis and treatment of human responses to actual or potential health problems" (1980a, p. 9). All entry-level registered nurses take the same national exam to achieve the RN credential. In order to gain eligibility to take the NCLEX–Registered Nurse (NCLEX-RN) examination, you may follow any of a variety of educational pathways.

Even though it can be expected that all RNs have a common minimum competency upon exit from a basic program and successful completion of the NCLEX-RN, it is important to understand the differences in the levels of educational preparation. Diploma, associate's degree, and bachelor's degree programs are designed to provide the education and clinical experience necessary for entry into the profession. Much debate exists about whether diploma and associate's degree nurses are technical nurses and whether professional nursing education isn't actually completed until the bachelor's degree, where entry into the profession should begin. Many nursing leaders believe that we should strive for differentiation of practice between the various levels of educational preparation.

Some programs allow a layperson to achieve a generic (first-degree) master's degree or a nursing doctorate (ND) before ever taking the NCLEX-RN exam. Advanced-practice nurses are educated as clinical specialists (CNS) or nurse practitioners (NP) or can have various other master's degrees and doctorates in nursing (Oermann, 1997). Upon graduation from any program of nursing, the first credential you may use is that of graduate nurse, or GN. This is a temporary designation that you may use until licensure or, in some cases, until you attempt the exam, whether or not you pass.

Diploma

The **diploma** program is probably the oldest form of nursing education. Its history is rich and long, with diploma schools prevalent by 1900 (Schwirian, 1998). Such a school is associated with a hospital, and in most cases the school concentrates the clinical portion of the program within that hospital. Diploma programs vary in length from 2 to 3 years.

These programs often provide a high ratio of clinical hours to class hours, with the number of nursing credits usually far exceeding the general education or liberal arts credits. Diploma schools thus provide a strong clinical-based education, which may translate into shorter orientation times in the work setting. Additionally, diploma graduates often have an acute-care background that helps them fill the needs of the hospital associated with the school. Even though diploma graduates may be well prepared to manage the care of their patients, they may not be as well prepared to manage or lead other nurses or peers.

Associate's Degree

In her 1951 doctoral dissertation, Mildred Montag described a type of nurse whose functional abilities were broader than a practical nurse's but narrower than a professional nurse's (Haase, 1990). Since their inception, **associate's degree** nursing programs have grown to comprise the majority of nursing programs nationwide (Haase, 1990; Schwirian, 1998). These programs are typically seated within community colleges. Their length is usually 2 years, 50% to 75% of which is focused on nursing science. The total number of credits required for an associate's degree is often approximately 70.

By far, associate's degree nursing programs offer the most common type of registered nurse preparation. The associate's degree nurse, considered the technical nurse, is well prepared to give comprehensive bedside patient care in the acute and long-term care settings. The associate's degree nurse is not as well prepared to take on management responsibilities or to practice in the home care or community health nursing environment. Often the lack of courses in critical care, community health nursing, and leadership and management, along with a host of general education requirements, separate the associate's degree nurse from the baccalaureate-prepared nurse.

Bachelor's Degree

In 1909 the first baccalaureate program in nursing was founded, within the school of medicine at the University of Minnesota (Schwirian, 1998). **Bachelor's degree** programs, based in colleges and universities, provide approximately 4 years of study. Typically, a bachelor's degree program requires approximately 120 credit hours, with about half dedicated to nursing courses. The remaining courses are in liberal arts and sciences.

A major difference between baccalaureate and diploma or associate's nursing education is the presence of management and leadership courses, which prepare the baccalaureate nurse for roles in these areas. The baccalaureate nurse often still requires the same, or perhaps slightly more, time to become comfortable with the technical skills of the patient care area but is often found to acclimate quickly to leadership responsibilities. In order to advance into leadership and other roles with a certain amount of autonomy, a nurse will need to earn a baccalaureate degree. If you prefer to progress to even more specialized and autonomous roles, you will find that a master's degree in nursing is required.

Master's Degree

Master's degree programs are highly specific and prepare students for advanced (very specialized and autonomous) nursing practice in a variety of settings. Registered nurses with master's degrees are found in such fields as higher education, staff development, and administration, as well as such careers as clinical specialist, consultant, nurse practitioner, and midwife. The length of a master's program ranges from 1 to 2 or more years, depending on the degree, certifications, and designations awarded (Schwirian, 1998).

Doctoral Degree

Doctoral degree programs prepare nurses to become the researchers, teachers, and clinicians who perpetuate and improve the art and science of nursing as a highly specialized profession. Doctoral programs often require at least 3 years of study beyond the master's degree level, a comprehensive examination, and a doctoral dissertation. The dissertation is a very rigorous process whereby the student engages in original research, guided by an advisory committee of accomplished faculty members. The research is supported through extensive literature review and presented in the form of a paper, often hundreds of pages in length.

Licensure
NCLEX-RN

The national licensure examination for registered nurses (NCLEX-RN) is planned and implemented by a group of experts within the National Council of State Boards of Nursing (NCSBN). The NCSBN recruits practicing nurses and provides experiential opportunities in item writing and reviewing skills. In this manner the NCSBN ensures that graduates who pass the licensing exam will be competent and safe as beginning practitioners.

The NCLEX-RN test plan is frequently updated and improved to reflect the nature of entry-level nursing practice. Panels of experts determine all characteristics of the exam. Item writers and reviewers are carefully chosen and trained. In April 1998 the test plan was implemented with two major updates:

1. Instead of considering the nursing process as a separate dimension to be tested, it was integrated throughout all areas of the examination.

2. The client-needs section was reordered and is now composed of the following categories: safe, effective care environment; health promotion and maintenance; psychosocial integrity; psychosocial integrity.

Each test taker is given a unique set of questions. Computer-based testing allows for this possibility. Each candidate is required to answer between 75 and 265 questions and has up to 5 hours to complete the examination. The faculty of your program is familiar with the current national licensing exam test plan and works diligently to ensure that upon graduation you are not only prepared to do well on the examination but also clearly prepared for safe, competent care at the entry level, including the ability to think critically and solve problems. To find out more about the national licensing exams, ask your faculty, call the NCSBN, or visit their website at www.ncsbn.org.

NCLEX-PN

The national licensure examination for practical or vocational nurses (NCLEX-PN) is planned and implemented by the NCSBN in a manner similar to that of the NCLEX-RN exam. The latest changes in the NCLEX-PN test plan, implemented in 1999, require that items address the cognitive level of analysis. Until 1999 such analysis was considered the domain of the RN.

Recent Licensure Changes

The recent changes in both the RN and the PN test plans, in addition to the higher levels of performance required for achievement of passing scores, will likely raise the bar for entry into nursing. To ensure the highest quality patient care as well as perpetuation of the profession, people seeking entry to the field must demonstrate competency reflecting the needs and expectations of a changing society. The student should take seriously every nursing program opportunity to gain knowledge and experience in preparation for successful performance on the licensing exam.

Scope of Practice

A nurse's **scope of practice** is defined by individual state nurse practice acts, which are part of the law or code governing that state; however, similarities exist between states. The individual state boards of nursing, which are located within varying government organizations at the state level, commonly exist to protect the consumers of nursing care by regulating the profession. The NCSBN is the unifying body for the state boards.

Licensed Practical Nursing

According to the ANA (1989), the practice of practical nursing is considered "directed" in that an LPN functions under the direction of an RN, physician, or other health care provider. Practical nurses are prepared to provide care in settings where patients are experiencing common health problems.

Registered Nursing

According to the ANA (1980b), the RN practices autonomously in a variety of health care settings, with patients in all stages of health and wellness throughout the age spectrum. Registered nursing practice requires specialized education and experience. The development of improvements in professional practice relies on nursing theory and research.

In the left column of Exercise 7-1, write your understanding of your scope of practice as an LPN. In the right column, relate your understanding of your future scope of practice as an RN.

Exercise 7-1

Scope of Practice as LPN	Scope of Practice as RN

Theories in Support of Nursing

According to Schwirian (1998), **nursing theory** is built upon several important adapted scientific theories:

Developmental, or Physiologic, Theories

Developmental theories teach nurses that all systems in the human body are interdependent. Many such theories help us understand the hows and whys of health and illness. For example, Maslow's Theory of the Hierarchy of Needs states that humans have certain basic needs, such as nutrition, hydration, shelter, and safety, that must be met before we can focus on more advanced, abstract needs, such as self-esteem or self-actualization (Taylor, Lillis, and LeMone, 2001). As nurses, we prioritize our care based on the basics needed to sustain life before we move on to other considerations. Multiple levels of needs may occur simultaneously, but a good rule to remember is that if the patient is unable to breathe, restoring the basic need takes priority over concerns over self-esteem.

Another developmental theory is Erikson's Theory of Psychosocial Development, which says that the six stages of psychosocial development are influenced by biologic, social, and environmental factors. The stages range from infancy, which Erikson labeled the stage of *trust versus mistrust*, through the lifespan to elder adulthood, labeled *ego integrity versus despair* (Erikson, 1980). According to this theory, humans, based on several influencing factors, experience either the positive or the negative aspect of each developmental stage, and we as nurses must adapt our care to the specific age and developmental stage in order to promote the person's positive development and overall health.

Systems Theory

Systems theory, principally developed by Ludwig von Bertallanaffy in the 1920s, defines the interdependence of environments in and around us. What this means for nursing is that we must understand that all parts of a system are connected, that a change in one part will have an effect on another. For instance, a person with low blood pressure will have multiorgan involvement. Similarly, if one person in a family is ill, then all members of that family will react to that illness. Systems theory can also be applied to organizations, groups, and professions. For instance, a change in the expected entry-level practice of new registered nurses may necessitate a change in the NCLEX-RN test plan, which will ripple to the faculty and to the students as well as to the consumer of nursing care.

Systems theory has identified the following fundamental concepts and characteristics of systems (Taylor, Lillis, and LeMone, 2001):

- The interrelated components act together toward the purpose of the whole.

- Because the components are arranged in a hierarchical structure and connected, a change in one component will necessarily ripple to other components, much like the effect of a pebble dropped into a pond.

- Systems have boundaries.

- Systems are both affected by and have an effect on the environment, both internally and externally.

Role Theory

Role theory helps you, as a nurse, function therapeutically in interactions and helps you understand behaviors in your patients, their families, and yourself. A role defines the expected behaviors of people in the particular role. Roles change over a lifetime, and at any one time a person may occupy several roles. This theory can be applied to you at this very moment. As you move from the role of practical nurse into that of registered nurse, you will experience role transition and possibly role confusion as you expand your nursing practice.

Adaptation Theory

Adaptation theory helps the nurse understand the ability of living things to adjust in response to internal and external stimuli. Adaptation occurs continuously, with input, output, and feedback loops. In studying adaptation theory, you can begin to understand how humans cope with stressors in these six dimensions: physical, developmental, emotional, intellectual, social, and spiritual (Potter and Perry, 1997).

Nursing Theorists

Many students enter their first theory classes with the predetermined idea that theory is only for faculty members and researchers and that everyday nurses do not need to know about it. However, nursing theory is the foundation upon which we base our practice as registered nurses. It is also the source from which new knowledge is generated, expanding and defining best practice and thereby improving outcomes for our patients. Every nurse must engage in evidence-based practice, that is, practice guided by diverse theories that help the nurse interpret the evidence and direct his or her decision making.

Numerous philosophies, models, and theories have built the foundation and expanded the knowledge unique to the profession. Most have in common four universal concepts that are central to nursing practice: person, health, environment, and nursing. These themes are described, defined, ordered, and interrelated in distinctive, meaningful, and powerful ways as nursing theorists endeavor to continue the development of nursing's unique body of knowledge. To discuss just a few theories without illustrating several more of them is difficult because they are in many cases interrelated, but for a beginning understanding, at least several major theorists and their works need to be briefly introduced.

FLORENCE NIGHTINGALE   Florence Nightingale, called "the Lady with the Lamp" for her ministrations to British soldiers during the Crimean War, determined in the 1850s that nursing knowledge was different from medical knowledge and that nursing duties should not include errands and chores, as was prevalent at the time, but rather focus only on the personal care of the patient. Nightingale believed that the nurse's job is to prepare the patient and the environment in such a way that nature could take its course. Nightingale believed that nursing required specialized education, and as a result of her convictions, she established a school for nurses in 1860. Modern nursing education has developed upon this foundation (Taylor, Lillis, and LeMone, 2001). Nightingale is also revered as one of the first nurse researchers and theorists, with the publication of her book *Notes on Nursing* in 1860. Unfortunately the profession did not accept the need for research and theory development until the 1950s (Alligood and Choi, 1998).

HILDEGARD E. PEPLAU   Hildegard E. Peplau was perhaps the first key contributor to the establishment of vital modern nursing theory, with the 1952 publication of her landmark book *Interpersonal Relations in Nursing*. Peplau determined that the only way nursing was going to make strides toward becoming an independent profession was for nurses to engage in scientific research. She believed that nursing research must grow out of and feed back to nursing practice. This work seemed to be the catalyst for nursing theory, igniting desire in many to build up the theoretical and scientific bases of nursing.

In the 1950s there was rampant, socially accepted discrimination against women, and nurses were strictly subservient to the physician; nursing was but a set of tasks. Peplau braved the waters and asserted that nursing should be an autonomous profession separate from practicing medicine and that the nurse's responsibility was to the patient. Peplau's theory is that the relationship between the nurse and the patient is central to nursing and that the interpersonal process that unfolds is therapeutic. The aim is to promote advancement of the patient's personality toward greater self-determination in life (Gastmans, 1998).

VIRGINIA HENDERSON   Virginia Henderson authored the *Textbook of the Principles and Practice of Nursing* (1955), which was the original resource for principles of nursing practice. Henderson may be more well known for the definition of nursing included in her text *Nature of Nursing* (1966), which states that nursing's primary responsibility is "to assist the individual, sick or well, in the performance of those activities contributing to the health or its recovery (or to a peaceful death) that he would perform unaided if he had the necessary strength, will or knowledge, and to do this in such a way as to help him gain independence as rapidly as possible" (p. 407).

Henderson is further credited with integrating the view of holism into nursing. She believed that humans have needs that are not only biologic but also psychologic, sociocultural, and spiritual. Based on these beliefs, she described 14 needs and inherent rights of the individual, which have served as an early yet enduring guide for nursing practice. These 14 fundamental elements are breathing, eating and drinking, eliminating, moving, sleeping and resting, selecting clothing and dressing, regulating body temperature, maintaining adequate hygiene, remaining free of harm and avoiding harming others, communicating, learning and seeking general fulfillment, having spirituality, working, and playing (Anderson, 1999; Taylor, Lillis, and LeMone, 2001).

DOROTHEA E. JOHNSON   Dorothea E. Johnson has created a theory, called the Behavioral Systems Model, that combines the essence of both developmental and systems theory (Johnson, 1980). She believes that a person is composed of seven interrelated behavioral components, which have basic requirements that nursing can help meet through comprehensive, individualized care:

- Attachment behaviors develop in infancy and continue throughout the lifespan. The ability to bond with another person is essential for gaining a sense of safety and belonging.

- Dependency behaviors allow others to care for or support the individual.

- Ingestive behaviors are related to nutrition and hydration, including issues of culture and society.

- Eliminative behaviors are related to body wastes as well as development of self-control in a variety of situations.

- Sexual behaviors are related to reproduction and sexual satisfaction, including issues of gender, culture, and society.

- Aggressive behaviors are related to protection of self or others.

- Achievement behaviors are related to the individual's mode of controlling the academic, corporeal, artistic, mechanical, and societal environments.

Johnson believes that nursing can help manipulate the external environment such that the individual is able to maintain balance, both internally and externally (Taylor, Lillis, and LeMone, 2001).

IMOGENE M. KING   Imogene M. King published her Interacting Systems Framework and Theory of Goal Attainment in 1981. King's scheme advances the concept that humans are composed of three interacting systems (personal, interpersonal, and social) that continually interact with the environment and are consequently changed. King proposes that through the interpersonal relationship of the nurse and patient, health can be achieved and maintained (relatively speaking). This theory has been since interpreted to include empathy as inherent within King's original interacting systems (Alligood, 2001).

MYRA E. LEVINE   Myra E. Levine supports the concept that nursing care is based on four principles of conservation:

1. Energy maintains the balance between factors that provide and those that expend the body's energy (i.e., nutrition, rest, and exertion).
2. Structural integrity promotes bodily healing.
3. Personal integrity promotes a sense of self and worth.
4. Social integrity promotes the social qualities of being.

Levine believes that all nursing actions are directed toward conservation in one or more of these areas (Taylor, Lillis, and LeMone, 2001).

DOROTHEA E. OREM   Dorothea E. Orem developed the Self-Care Deficit Theory of Nursing, which is based on the belief that humans have an internal drive to care for themselves. The outcome of all nursing actions should be to promote the capacity for self-care in all individuals. Orem defines activities of self-care as purposeful, ordered, and derived from the experiences of daily life. The degree to which a person is able to participate in this is called *self-care agency*. In contrast, *self-care deficit* is the degree to which the patient is unable to perform self-care. Orem proposed three self-care requisites, or areas of need, in order to maintain self-care:

1. Universal self-care needs are the basics required by everyone in support of life and health, such as air, nutrition, hydration, elimination, rest, exercise, privacy, community, and safety.
2. Developmental needs make for an environment supportive of human development.
3. Health deviation calls for measures to diagnose illness or injury and reestablish health.

Orem further divides self-care needs into levels based on degree of patient participation and control. At the wholly compensatory level, the nurse meets all the needs of the patient. At the partly compensatory level, the nurse and patient manage care together. At the supportive-educative level, the patient has control and manages care with little assistance.

MARTHA E. RODGERS   Martha E. Rodgers created the multifaceted Theory of Unitary Human Beings in the 1950s. This theory, based on the research and work of numerous other disciplines, espoused recognition that human beings are the purpose for nursing. Rogers asserted that both humans and the environment are composed of energy fields that are continually interacting. Rodgers further declared that human action becomes predictable through scrutiny of the characteristic changes in the energy fields.

SISTER CALLISTA ROY   Sister Callista Roy developed the Theory of Adaptation, which is considered a fundamental philosophy for many nursing programs around the world. The four basic assumptions of the Roy Model of Adaptation are as follows:

1. Each human being is an individual with biologic, psychologic, and social needs and stressors.
2. Individuals use both intrinsic and learned coping mechanisms to adapt to stressors. Adaptive responses, which can be either positive or negative, are influenced by factors associated both with the stressor and with prior experience.
3. Four areas stimulate the adaptation response: physiologic, self-concept, interdependent behaviors, and role/function.
4. An individual moves back and forth across the health-illness continuum based on the success of the adaptive responses.

Roy believes that nursing is a major social force in the world and that enhancing the health, welfare, and safety of all is nursing's mission.

BETTY NEUMAN Betty Neuman created the Healthcare Systems Model, which states that a person is a complex system that responds to stressors originating in both the internal and external environments. Each individual's response is unique and must be treated uniquely. The Healthcare Systems Model guides nursing practice within three levels of prevention:

1. At the primary level, nurses are engaged in health promotion and illness prevention.
2. The secondary level deals with treatment of symptoms.
3. At the tertiary level, nurses facilitate rehabilitation and strengthening of internal and external resources to prevent further insult.

Neuman's model is also widely accepted as an organizing framework for nursing care.

JEAN WATSON Jean Watson's Theory of Transpersonal Care (1988) supports the concept that nursing provides humanistic, holistic care, which is the art, science, and moral standard of nursing. The provision of transpersonal care is based on 10 "carative factors," which serve to promote health and prevent illness: values, faith and hope, compassion for self and others, trusting, rapport, encouraging and accepting emotional expression, analytic decision making, collaborative teaching and learning, supportive environment, and meeting needs.

Exercise 7-2

Examples	Former LPN Role Application	Future RN Role Application

OTHER THEORISTS   Many other theorists have contributed to the body of nursing knowledge that we claim today, each deserving of celebration. These include Madeline Leininger, Joyce Fitzpatrick, Lydia Hall, Rosemarie Rizzo Parse, and Ide Jean Orlando. Although more theorists are not mentioned in this text, the student should seek out and understand the development of nursing theory and its influence on the nursing practice of the present and future. "To improve education and practice through theory is possible only when the profession accepts the reality that nursing theories are not written in stone ... There is much theorizing left to do and practitioners are needed to identify it" (Levine, 1995, p. 14). Bringing theory and research into practice and subsequently conducting new research will create the practices that will ultimately improve patient care best.

In Exercise 7-2, consider how the nursing theories within this chapter can be applied to your daily practice. Provide examples, and explain how they apply to your former role as an LPN and your future role as an RN.

Summary

In this chapter you have begun exploring the differences between the licensed practical nurse and the registered nurse. The educational preparation and licensure of the roles are similar in process yet different in content and practice. The LPN has attended school for approximately 1 year, including both nursing classes and clinicals. The LPN serves the client in a directed and limited role. In contrast, the RN attends school from 2 to 4 years, composed of nursing classes, clinicals, and liberal arts and sciences. The RN serves the client in both autonomous and collaborative roles.

Critical Thinking Questions

1. A 46-year-old male is admitted to your unit after experiencing a stroke. He is a professional potter, he has 4-year-old and 18-year-old sons, and his wife is a teacher who is also working on her master's degree. In his role as a potter, he is also the primary home caregiver. He has a strong family history of cardiovascular disease and had ignored signs and symptoms of hypertension before having the stroke. He has left-sided weakness and is experiencing expressive aphasia.

   a. What are the potential patient concerns?

   b. What problems may the patient face?

   c. How will the patient's stroke potentially affect other systems within his body?

    d. What further assessment questions do you need to ask before formulating a plan of care?

2. In your new role as an RN, you will be working with other RNs who may have obtained their licenses through a different educational path than you. One often misunderstands or even belittles a different educational pathway when looking at it from the path that he or she took. What measures can you use to understand the strengths of the nurses with whom you work?

3. As an RN you will be required to delegate tasks to LPNs on your team. Identify a delegated situation in your past LPN experience that might have caused a strain on the boundaries of your LPN role.

    a. Knowing the limitations of your LPN role and having learned more about your new RN role, what were the potential consequences to your completion of the task assigned to you?

    b. What were the consequences?

    c. What were the outcomes of the situation? How did you feel afterwards?

References

Alligood MR: Research corner: a theory of nursing empathy in King's Interacting Systems, *Tenn Nurse* 64(2):18, 2001.

Alligood MR, Choi EC: Evolution of nursing theory development. In Marriner-Tomey A, Alligood MR, editors: *Nursing theorists and their work*, ed 4, St Louis, 1998, Mosby.

American Nurses Association: *Nursing: a social policy statement*, Kansas City, Mo, 1980a, Author.

American Nurses Association: *The nursing practice act: suggested state legislation*, Kansas City, Mo, 1980b, Author.

American Nurses Association: *Entry-level competencies of graduates of educational programs in practical nursing*, Kansas City, Mo, 1989, Author.

Anderson M: Virginia Avenel Henderson: a modern legend, *Wyo Nurses Newsl* 12(1):9, 1999.

Erikson EH: *Identity and the life cycle*. New York, 1980, Norton.

Gastmans C: Interpersonal relations in nursing: a philosophical-ethical analysis of the work of Hildegard E. Peplau, *J Adv Nurs* 28(6):1312, 1998.

Haase PT: *The origins and rise of Associate degree nursing*. Durham, NC, 1990, Duke University Press.

Henderson V: *The nature of nursing: a definition and its implications for practice, research, and education*. New York, 1966, MacMillan.

Johnson D: The Behavioral System Model of Nursing. In Riehl JP, Roy C, editors: *Conceptual models for nursing practice*, ed 2, New York, 1980, Appleton-Century-Crofts.

Levine ME: The rhetoric of nursing theory, *Image J Nurs Sch* 27(1):11, 1995.

Nightingale F: *Notes on nursing: what it is and what it is not*. New York, 1860, D. Appleton & Co.

Oermann MH: *Professional nursing practice*, Stamford, Conn, 1997, Appleton & Lange.

Peplau H: *Interpersonal relations in nursing*. New York, 1952, Putnam.

Potter P, Perry A: *Fundamentals of nursing: concepts, process, and practice*, St Louis, 1997, Mosby.

Schwirian PM: *Professionalization of nursing: current issues and trends,* ed 3, Philadelphia, 1998, Lippincott.

Taylor C, Lillis C, LeMone P: *Fundamentals of nursing: the art and science of nursing care,* ed 4, Philadelphia, 2001, Lippincott.

Watson J: *Nursing: human science and human care—a theory of nursing.* New York, 1988, National League for Nursing.

Section 4

Care Planner versus Care Giver: Distinguishing the Roles

Chapter 8

Understanding the Nursing Process

Key Terms

actual problem
assessment
critical pathway
cues
identifying criteria
implementation
interview
introduction phase
nursing diagnosis

nursing process
objective data
observation
physical assessment
potential problem
subjective data
termination phase
validating
working phase

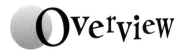Overview

The **nursing process** is a critical concept necessary for the provision of optimal nursing care, the clear understanding of which is the outcome priority of this chapter. The application of nursing process theory in daily practice is what sets nursing apart from other health care disciplines. In this chapter you first learn about the evolution of the nursing process concept. The chapter then introduces you to the six steps involved in the nursing process: assessment, diagnosis, outcome identification, planning, implementation, and evaluation (FYI 8-1).

Historical Perspective

The term *nursing process* dates back to 1955, when Lydia Hall first identified the practice of nursing as having three distinct steps: making observations, giving care, and validating. In 1967 the Western Interstate Commission for Higher Education (WICHE) published a definition of the nursing process that was theoretically different from anything before or since, focusing on the interaction between the patient and the nurse. This resulted in a four-step nursing process based on communication, rather than just nursing action and client response (Craven and Hirnle, 2000).

In 1967 Yura and Walsh developed a four-step nursing process that became the foundation for the problem-solving process familiar to modern-day nurses, including assessment, planning, implementation, and evaluation (Craven and Hirnle, 2000). The American Nurses Association (ANA) added a fifth item to the nursing process concept in 1973, when diagnosis was distinguished as a separate functional step. **Nursing diagnosis** quickly became a central theme of study for nursing theorists, and in 1980 actual and potential nursing diagnoses were considered essential to practice.

The study of the nursing process continues to advance and refine nursing practice. In 1991 the ANA added yet another chapter to the book of nursing innovation by introducing outcome identification as a new step in the nursing process (Craven and Hirnle, 2000). The six steps of the nursing process as it is now known include assessment, diagnosis, outcome identification, planning, implementation, and evaluation. The nursing

FYI 8-1   LPN and RN Roles in the Nursing Process

Phase of Nursing Process	LPN Role	RN Role
Assessment	Gather basic objective and subjective data to be analyzed by the RN	Complete and analyze a comprehensive assessment of the patient within the physiologic, psychologic, social, cultural, and spiritual realms
Diagnosis	Understand the diagnoses the RN has assigned and what that means for the patient's plan of care	Cluster assessment cues into relevant groups of identifying criteria and formulate individualized nursing diagnoses
Planning	Clearly understand the priorities and interventions identified in the plan of care that are the LPN's responsibility	Prioritize nursing diagnoses and individual interventions to be carried out by the health care team
Implementation	Carry out specified interventions as directed by the RN	Direct and carry out nursing interventions, participation in the implementation of collaborative interventions, and to follow up on those interventions appropriately delegated to other members of the health care team
Evaluation	Provide the RN with basic assessment data that reflects measures indicated in the plan of care	Comprehensively evaluate the patient progress toward achievement of outcomes and to adjust the plan of care accordingly

Exercise 8-1

My roles in the nursing process involve:

process is often referred to as nursing's problem-solving method. In many ways it is similar to the scientific method.

Take this time to assess what you believe your roles to be in the nursing process by completing the statement in Exercise 8-1.

Nursing Process

Assessment

The first step of the nursing process is **assessment**, which involves the collection of both objective and subjective data about an individual, family, or community. You need to examine five realms to thoroughly complete assessment: physiologic, psychologic, social, cultural, and spiritual. You must survey each realm for factors that may affect the patient's health status. If you concentrate on only one or two areas, you will likely miss important data, make inappropriate nursing diagnoses, and carry out inappropriate or incomplete nursing actions.

The RN must gather data from many areas, along with information about the patient's current and past health concerns. A thorough health history is completed upon the patient's admission into the health care setting or at the first interaction of the patient (or significant other) and the nurse. The history is obtained either through the primary source (the patient), through a secondary source (those who know the patient, such as family, friends), or through the patient's past medical record. The history often contains valuable insights into what is currently happening or what may happen concerning the patient's health.

The nurse must understand that every time he or she interacts with the patient in any way, assessment is taking place. While the nursing process as a whole may seem elaborate or confusing to the beginner, part of what the new RN comes to understand is that the nursing process is so integral to minute-to-minute practice that it often occurs without notice. The process behind nursing practice requires a whole new way of thinking, which soon becomes second nature. This manner of thought is likely not uncommon to adult students who must make critical decisions in everyday life. What is likely to be different is that the nurse must have the ability to keep multiple patients' many problems and requisite assessments, interventions, and evaluations in mind concurrently, all the while planning for what comes next for every patient. Although assessment may become second nature, the nurse must still think carefully and deeply about it. Because assessment is carried out every time the patient is seen, it becomes as natural as breathing, and no less important. However, the level of rigorous and meticulous care in managing the assessment makes the difference.

Assessment is accomplished through a number of mechanisms. The nurse observes the patient and the surrounding situation, interviews both primary and secondary sources, examines the patient from head to toe in a systematic manner, and interprets laboratory data. The RN's assessment will contain both objective and subjective data. **Objective data** is information that is observed and leaves little room for interpretation, facts that can be measured and verified. Examples of objective data are vital signs, size and location of a wound, color of drainage, or any assessment that does not require personal perspective or opinion to document.

Subjective data is information experienced and described only by the patient and cannot be verified as to its characteristics or easily quantified. Examples of subjective data include such feelings and experiences as the patient's pain, fear, nausea, and uneasiness. In instances of subjective data collection, the best practice is always to write exactly what the patient says, using quotation marks, rather than paraphrase, which is when the RN documents in his or her own words what the patient has said. Be careful not to use your own opinion words, just the facts.

DATA COLLECTION METHODS   Data collection is accomplished by several different methods, including interview, observation, and physical assessment.

The **interview** is a dialogue or question-and-answer session with the patient or people accompanying the patient. Through interview you obtain the complete nursing history, which includes demographics; the chief complaint, normal health-seeking behaviors, current state of health, and medications; and developmental, social, environmental, and family history. You may wish to interview the patient and the significant other separately for verification of data and to gain perspective on a particular situation, or the patient may desire to be interviewed alone. In each case, provide as much privacy as possible, remembering that voices easily penetrate the curtain drawn around the bed. During the interview, seat yourself at the same level as the interviewee. Keep in mind that the patient may be tired or in pain and not able to talk for long periods of time.

The three distinct phases of the interview process are as follows:

1. During the **introduction phase** the nurse gives his or her name and credentials as well as the role to be played in the life of the patient for the immediate future. The patient should know what to expect and understand what is expected of him or her. This is the time to create the impression of compassion and competence. Ask the patient what additional comfort measures you might provide before beginning. The patient has the right to understand how the information will be recorded and who will have access to it. If possible, record information directly onto the assessment form during the interview.
2. During the **working phase** of the interview, the nurse predominantly collects subjective data, whose quality and quantity is highly dependent on the interviewing skills of the nurse. Therapeutic communication techniques will likely improve the value of the data you gather. Some techniques to remember are to maintain eye contact, listen closely, ask appropriate questions and repeat the patient's words to verify understanding, use open-ended questions that require more than yes-or-no answers, and let the patient do the talking.
3. The **termination phase**, the final stage of the interview, is when the nurse summarizes what has been learned and verifies with the patient that all relevant information has been documented. Before exiting, inform the patient about when you will return and what can be expected to happen next. Ask about any other questions the patient may have and any comfort measures you might provide before leaving the area.

Observation is the collection of data through seeing, listening, smelling, touching, and generally sensing the patient and the immediate environment as well as the larger context of the situation.

Physical assessment is the collection of objective data through inspection, auscultation, palpation, and percussion. The nursing physical assessment differs from the medical physical assessment by determining functional abilities and deficits in order to focus the plan of care and help identify the outcome priorities.

The nurse must individualize and prioritize the nursing assessment according to each patient situation. The assessment will have different perspectives and focuses with pediatrics compared with adults and from one setting to another. At other times the nurse must complete targeted or emergency assessments only.

ORGANIZATION OF DATA COLLECTION   Nursing assessments must be organized in a clear, systematic manner that permits logical progression of the data. Organization of the data promotes accurate and comprehensive determination of the plan of care and subsequent prioritization of nursing interventions. Furthermore, clearly documented nursing assessments are valuable tools for communicating and collaborating with other members of the health care team in the provision of total patient care.

VALIDATING ASSESSMENT DATA   **Validating**, or verifying, assessment data is necessary to ensure accuracy. Be alert to instances where what the patient is stating is markedly different from what you are observing or when specific measurable data lack initial objectivity. Methods of data validation range from repeating back what you believe you understand of the patient's story for clarification, to asking another nurse to check a suspicious vital sign or interpret a 6-second telemetry strip.

EXAMPLE OF GATHERED ASSESSMENT DATA   A patient with type II diabetes mellitus is admitted to the hospital because of necrosis of his left great toe, secondary to poor circulation. The patient is noted to have decreased dorsalis pedal and posterior-tibial pulses in the left foot. The foot and ankle have a mottled appearance, and the skin is dry and shiny. The characteristic lack of hair of the lower extremities is suggestive of long-standing peripheral vascular disease. The patient states that there is pain in the left foot and leg and is scheduled for surgery to remove the great toe and surrounding involved tissue. The overall outcome priority is to provide an environment that will optimize the surgical intervention, while establishing a level of comfort and safety that promotes a return to a level of function higher than the current level of wellness.

Diagnosis

The clustering of **cues**, or data points, gathered in the assessment phase helps define the care priorities and the associated "problems," or nursing diagnoses. Every nursing diagnosis must be substantiated by **identifying criteria**, also known as defining characteristics. For a nursing diagnosis to be accepted, often numerous signs and symptoms together make up the actual diagnosis. These identifying criteria must be present in the patient in order to assign that diagnosis. Caution and attention to detail are crucial here because many diagnoses are similar but have different interventions and different outcomes, and patients will almost always have multiple diagnoses.

Diagnoses may be either actual or potential. An **actual problem** or diagnosis is substantiated by the patient's current signs and symptoms. This problem is identified as requiring specialized nursing interventions or collaborative interventions from the rest of the health care team.

A **potential problem** or diagnosis is understood by the nurse as likely to develop although not currently evidenced in the signs and symptoms. Potential problems require the nurse to be vigilant in planning care so that actual problems are avoided.

One of the mistakes of the beginning nurse is to identify patient problems without supporting data. Also, the beginning nurse might identify potential problems but give supporting data for actual problems. In either case, the nurse must take care to use data correctly to individualize the plan of care.

Nursing diagnoses are written in a format that places the problem as related to an etiology, or cause or source, of the problem. At this point some schools add the "as evidenced by" statement. The identifying criteria or defining characteristics follow as evidence that this problem or diagnosis is substantiated by assessed signs and symptoms.

Continuation of the earlier diabetes example will provide insight to diagnosis development. The nurse has gathered the following data: (1) patient's complaint of pain in the left foot; (2) 1+ pedal and dorsalis pedis pulses; (3) foot temperature cool to touch; (4) great toe dry, black appearance, with no nail noted, and second toe with a 2 cm diameter black area; and (5) decreased sensation of the foot. Additional information gathered from the history reveals a decrease in eyesight as a result of bilateral cataracts and a decrease in hearing.

From these data the following actual problems can be identified. The patient has pain in the left foot, which is an actual problem and is written as such. Pain, actual, related to the complications of the disease process, as evidenced by the patient's subjective account of pain in the left foot, visible limping, and guarding of the area upon assessment. Potential problems are related to the patient's failing eyesight and hearing, which may compromise the patient's ability to respond to an unfamiliar environment, causing injury. Therefore the patient is at risk for injury, and the problem statement is written: "High risk for injury, related to failing eyesight, decreased hearing, and unfamiliar surroundings." No evidence exists that this is an actual injury that has already occurred, yet the problem statement will alert nurses to be extra vigilant in patient care. The assessment process requires identifying and ordering cues to determine the level of care needed to identify patient problems and outcome priorities. Many institutions continue to use the North American Nursing Diagnosis Association's (NANDA, 2001) list of standard nursing diagnoses in the development of the plan of care (see Appendix C for a list of NANDA nursing diagnoses). Much argument exists regarding standardized nursing diagnoses in the planning of care; however, some opponents claiming that such diagnoses promote a failure to individualize the plan of care for each patient.

You may need to make clarifications when collaborating with other health care workers on a patient's plan of care. For example, you as a nurse would diagnose a patient with hypoxemia as having "ineffective tissue perfusion." However, you would need to communicate to a respiratory therapist the patient's need for a respiratory treatment. This communication will include specific signs and symptoms with which the patient is presenting, rather than the nursing diagnosis. A common health care language may soon be developed to identify problems and implement collaborative plans of care more clearly.

The plan of care includes independent, dependent, and collaborative interventions, which are coordinated by RNs. Evaluation of the plan of care is also the responsibility of RNs, using data collected from many sources, including licensed practical nurses and unlicensed assistive personnel. RNs direct the data collection process and implementation of the interventions through delegation of duties to the resources available to them. The determination of the plan's effectiveness includes the evaluation of the team effort in carrying out the plan. Decisions regarding changes in the plan will be the RNs' responsibility.

Outcome Identification

Whether using NANDA or another reference when identifying problem areas and building the plan of care, the nurse must identify the criteria for evaluating the intervention outcomes. Every diagnosis is associated with specific, individualized expected outcomes or goals. These expectations must be measurable and clearly communicated, along with signs of attainment or nonattainment and dates and times for evaluation. Precise articulation of the expected outcome criteria will ensure that each nurse or team member assessing the patient will be looking for the same clues, which may signal a need for a change in the plan of care or reevaluation of the outcome priority.

Measurability means that the outcome can be consistently evaluated. An example of a measurable goal would be that the patient be able to ambulate 50 feet by a certain date and 100 feet by a certain later date. As another example, an outcome identification may be related to the goal of decreasing a patient's infection. Two measurable outcome criteria would be "no elevated temperature, and WBCs within normal range." Any nurse caring for the patient on the day designated for evaluation of the outcome will know by what measures the patient has attained or failed to attain the outcome and will adjust the plan of care accordingly.

Planning

The plan of care, developed during the planning phase of the nursing process, includes the process of identifying the interventions needed for the patient to regain a level of independence at or higher than he or she had before admission into the health care setting. Inherent to the planning process is prioritization of the nursing diagnoses as well as the collaborative patient care issues. This process is often simultaneous with the actual development of the diagnoses and outcomes. RNs will likely be compelled into action by prioritizing the urgent issues.

Establishment of the outcome priority is a planning mechanism. This concept may help the beginning RN understand that optimal nursing care involves constant assessment and reevaluation of the plan of care and substantiation of the outcome priority at any given moment. Planning involves the setting of both short-term and long-term goals or outcomes (Smeltzer and Bare, 2000). This substep often occurs when identifying outcome criteria. Short-term goals are outcomes that are likely, or required, to be achieved in the acute setting before discharge to a subacute setting is permitted. Long-term goals are outcomes that, although they are being addressed, are not likely to be achieved until some later time in a nonacute setting.

A serious element of planning patient care is determining whether the RN can legally order the nursing care that the patient requires. Here the RN is accountable to ensure that appropriate medical and ancillary interventions are prescribed and carried out in a collaborative manner. Knowing what you can and cannot do autonomously as an RN is imperative to safe, full practice.

Planning ultimately involves mapping out specific, individualized nursing actions that aim to achieve the desired outcomes associated with the nursing diagnoses. To appropriately plan interventions, the RN must consider all aspects of the patient, including age, culture, gender, and past experiences with health care. Planning includes ensuring that ethical and established standards of practice be maintained. Interventions should extend beyond the patient to include the environment and family unit. Including such context as the larger patient situation is essential to complete planning (Smeltzer and Bare, 2000).

In some institutions for one of the most common and predictable diagnoses, a **critical pathway** may be initiated. This is a plan of care that assists RNs in defining, within time frames, the expected level of care needed, some specific nursing and medical interventions, and the evaluation intervals. Critical pathways for many diagnoses are developed from patient norms within a particular health care concern and are often specific to the facility, unit, and even physician. They are effective tools for nurses to use as guides, but you must be alert for patient problems that fall out of the pathway and need to receive individualized attention.

Implementation

Implementation, the carrying out of the plan of care, requires a multidisciplinary approach. Licensed practical nurses collect data, implement actions specific to the patient care needs, administer basic teaching, record data as well as interventions, and report to RNs the progress the patient is making. RNs are responsible for delegating and coordinating the care that is given, implementing advanced interventions, evaluating and updating the plan of care and the associated outcome priorities, and engaging in and documenting patient and family education. The RN serves as gatekeeper and all-around organizer of all care and interventions that the multidisciplinary health care team provides. Accountability for both independent and interdependent functions remains a part of the role of the RN. As interventions are administered and completed, evaluation becomes an ever-present and crucial part of the role.

Evaluation

Evaluation is the process of examining the effectiveness of the plan of care and adjusting it to ultimately meet the needs of the patient. Outcome achievement is also determined as part of the evaluation. Assessment and evaluation occur simultaneously and continually. Unique, inventive changes in the plan of care come about as necessary when RNs use their critical thinking skills as part of the evaluation process. LPNs assist in the evaluation process by reporting progress and assessment data promptly

Exercise 8-2

As an LPN, my current responsibilities regarding the nursing process include:

In my new role as an RN, my responsibilities regarding the nursing process will include:

and accurately. The RN interprets the data and adjusts the plan of care to best meet the patient's needs. An appropriate plan of care may require no changes if the patient's condition is progressing as expected.

Now that you have studied the chapter, complete the sentences in Exercise 8-2.

Summary

The nursing process has evolved over many years from a three-step model to a six-step model of assessment, diagnosis, outcome identification, planning, implementation, and evaluation. The complex task of creating an individualized plan of care is crucial to the role of the RN. The RN retains full accountability for ensuring that the plan of care is carried out in a sensitive and effective manner. Meticulous attention is paid to assessment and evaluation to ensure that from minute to minute, all patient needs are anticipated, identified, and being met.

Critical Thinking Questions

1. For the following scenarios, what are the identified nursing diagnosis or problem statements?

   a. An 8 year old, newly diagnosed as an insulin-dependent diabetic, will be going home.

   b. A 72 year old with COPD, recovering from pneumonia, currently on 2 L of oxygen per nasal cannula, with a pulse oximeter reading between 90% and 94%. The patient becomes dyspneic and tachycardic while getting up to use the bathroom and returns to baseline after 10 minutes' rest.

c. A 24-year-old female in her third trimester of pregnancy with pan-edema, and blood pressure of 150/88 mm Hg and 160/99 mm Hg on two occasions 4 hours apart. She complains of not being able to get her rings off and of a headache.

d. A newborn is in the first 24 hours of birth and before going home.

2. For the following situations, what assessment questions would you need to ask?

a. You complete an 0700 blood sugar reading on your patient and get a level of 265.

b. You get a blood pressure reading of 190/110 mm Hg on an individual who is attending a wellness fair.

c. The health care aide reports that a patient, admitted to your unit to rule out GI bleed, just had a 100 ml emesis.

d. You walk into a room to do an assessment on your patient and find him sitting on the floor next to the bed.

e. After waking your patient you assess your patient's lungs and find fine crackles bilaterally in the bases.

f. You are assessing a 6-year-old patient who has just had a full liquid dinner, and you note that the patient is blue around the lips.

3. You are scheduled to discharge a patient home. The patient has an ongoing problem identified as "decreased tissue perfusion, peripheral r/t vascular changes of diabetes, and as evidenced by pulse per Doppler only, complaint of cold feet, pain, numbness, and tingling to the toes. The patient has had a femoral-popliteal bypass and now has 1+ pedal pulses bilaterally." Design a discharge plan of care, including the necessary teaching that will need to be done.

References

American Nurses Association Congress for Practice: *Standards of practice.* Washington, DC, 1973, Author.

Craven RF, Hirnle CJ: *Fundamentals of nursing: human health and function,* ed 3, Philadelphia, 2000, Lippincott.

North American Nursing Diagnosis Association: *NANDA nursing diagnoses: definitions and classifications, 2001-2002.* Philadelphia, 2001, Author.

Smeltzer SC, Bare BG: *Brunner and Suddarth's textbook of medical-surgical nursing,* Philadelphia, 2000, Lippincott.

Yura H, Walsh MB: *The nursing process: assessing, planning, implementing, and evaluating.* The proceedings of the Continuing Education Series conducted at the Catholic University of America. Washington, DC, 1967, Catholic University of America Press.

Chapter 9

The RN as a Critical Thinker

Key Terms

assumption
available information
clinical judgment
concepts
consequences
creativity
critical thinking
cultivated thinking
curiosity
deductive reasoning

implications
inductive reasoning
inference
intuitive thought
point of view
purpose
question at issue
rational thought
reasoned thought
reflection

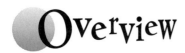verview

As you transition to the role of RN, it becomes more and more important to make sound clinical decisions based on your knowledge, experience, and skill. Thinking critically is a skill that you learn and hone throughout your nursing program and subsequent career. Critical thinking is purposeful and rational and sets out to accomplish a specified goal (Paul, 1995). The only way to become a critical thinker is to learn the process and practice.

This chapter explores many aspects of critical thinking, such as its practical application to nursing. The elements of critical thought as well as attributes of the critical thinker are presented. Situations requiring the RN to think critically and anticipate the associated outcomes are presented.

Definition of Critical Thinking

Critical thinking has been described in many ways, such as a way of knowing, a habit of mind, a rational process of thought, and a scientific process (Boychuk Duchscher, 1999). It is considered a skill that is necessary in the nursing process. Gordon (2000) found several definitions for critical thinking. For the purposes of this text, the following definition is offered: **critical thinking** is a purposeful, goal-directed process of inquiry that utilizes available facts, principles, theories, and abstractions to analyze, make inferences, solve problems, or arrive at decisions. This definition is operational, meaning that it has a base in practice and that implications exist for nurses within their scope of practice (Figure 9-1).

Purpose of Critical Thinking

All individuals think. Each time we engage in a decision-making process, we have an intended outcome in mind. However, we make decisions every day that do not lead to the expected or intended outcomes. How often have we decided to purchase a product based on what we have heard in commercials, only to be disappointed in the product after using it? Our decision might have become biased by the emotion of buying the product

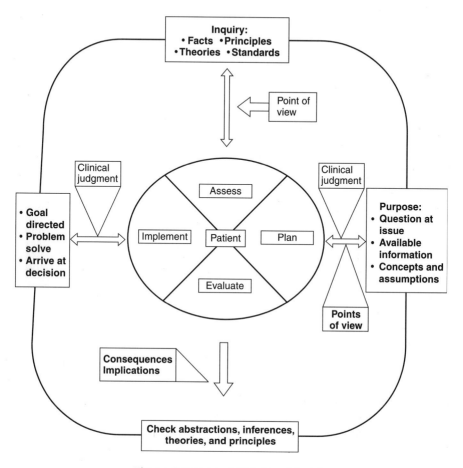

Figure 9-1 Critical Thinking Model.

or by the carefully crafted bravado of the advertising firm. If we had researched the product by other means before giving in to our impulses and purchasing it, we might have discovered general consumer dissatisfaction in the item, and our choice might have been different.

We assume that every nurse wants the health care consumer, the patient, to receive the best care possible. The nurse makes multiple decisions on a daily basis that will affect the patient's outcomes. The nurse must make these decisions using a critical thinking process. Complete Exercise 9-1, answering the questions related to critical thinking.

Exercise 9-1

List words you would use to define critical thinking:

List the characteristics of a nurse who you believe to be an expert:

Describe in detail a situation that demonstrates this nurse's expertise:

When telling the story, how many of the words you listed as defining critical thinking did you use?

What additional words have come to mind now that you have told the story?

Need for Critical Thinking

Hansten and Washburn (1999) indicate that the nurse must be able to think critically as a way to decrease errors, sentinel events, and assist in cultivating an improved patient care system. The nurse needs to give careful, complex consideration into what must be done and how best to do it (Greenwood 2000). This conscious effort is facilitated though a critical thought process. Boychuk Duchscher (1999) reports that as nursing is guided by theoretical concepts, the process of inquiry into these concepts is applied through critical thought. Furthermore, the process of evaluating nursing care occurs through critical thought. The nurse should challenge his or her own previously established thoughts and labels. An insightful, reflective thought process distinguishes the nurse as a careful thinker.

Types of Reasoning Embedded in Critical Thinking

Reasoned Thought

Reasoned thought is discriminating and prudent and does not allow emotion, feelings, or prejudices to skew decisions. Individuals who practice reasoned thought recognize when negative factors may be interfering with their ability to think clearly. The practice of reasoned thought is an intricate part of the critical thinking process.

Clinical Judgment

Clinical judgment is perceptive understanding of a situation based on knowledge, empirical data (data that can be observed or experienced), theory, and scientific inquiry (see Figure 9-1). Clinical judgment requires a series of decisions based on changing observations and collected data. "Clinical judgment is the complex cognitive process by which a clinician interprets patient behaviors and builds a communicable description of the status of the patient" (Chase, 1995, p. 154). Through clinical judgment the nurse makes decisions on whether to proceed with or revise a course of action. The inquiry (investigational or exploratory) subprocess necessary for sound clinical judgment is critical thinking.

The nursing process emerges as the framework for the RN to design care based on the inquiry process. The standard of care dictates that the nurse assess, analyze, plan, implement, and evaluate a plan of care for each patient. Careful thought is continually given to the process to expose faults. Critical thinking sets the standard for careful thought, and careful thought must be the practice standard for the nurse.

Nursing care is becoming research based and guided by theory and practice standards. As nursing requires a more scientific approach, the RN must become more knowledgeable in regard to following standards of care. The RN role, which involves collaboration with physicians and other health care providers, is more autonomous in nature than that of LPN. The complexity of the current health care environment requires more carefully prepared nurses, nurses who can think clearly, carefully, and purposefully. The nurse who can think critically is better prepared for the increasing demands of his or her responsibilities.

Experience, knowledge, and skills are required in order to think critically (Paul, 1995). Critical thought is a disciplined, rational, and self-directed activity that uses standards and criteria (Paul, 1995; Paul, Elder, and Bartell, 1997). Critical thought assists the nurse in making more effective clinical decisions. The nurse who engages in critical thought will meet more of the patient's needs and effect positive patient outcomes.

Related Thinking Skills

Many related thinking skills support the critical thinking process, such as cultivated thinking, and deductive and inductive reasoning.

Cultivated Thinking

People who engage in critical thought can be said to practice **cultivated thinking**, which is organized, enlightened, and educated. By organizing the thought process, the individual is able to make sense of information. Relevant data are sorted and prioritized in a coherent manner. The nurse uses the nursing process to gather assessments and cluster relevant data in order to identify actual and potential patient problems.

The cultivated thinker does not assume that he or she has gathered all the pertinent information yet. The cultivated thinker is not arrogant and recognizes traits that interfere with the ability to gain knowledge. This type of thinker seeks the latest and best information available to make the most appropriate decisions. The RN who continues to update the data and stay well informed will best meet the patients' needs.

Deductive Reasoning

The nurse must logically analyze situations every day, and how this is done demonstrates the ability to solve problems. Collection of data, part of the assessment phase of the nursing process, is followed by analysis to formulate a plan of care. The process of going from broad information to specific details, or general to specific, is **deductive reasoning**. Taking general assessment data, drawing conclusions, identifying problems or needs, and formulating a plan of care is a deductive reasoning process. The nursing process is an example of deductive reasoning since it involves taking data and deducing a plan of care.

Specific data lead to specific nursing diagnoses. The North American Nursing Diagnosis Association (NANDA) provides the standard nursing diagnoses for nurses to follow. Standard nursing diagnoses require specific assessment data to support their use. The nurse who uses deductive reasoning sets out to prove the result through supporting data. The data will likely measure and describe a physical or psychological problem that interferes with the patient's ability to satisfactorily perform activities of daily living. The problem usually also implies a need for assistance with the activity.

For example, a patient has a problem that prevents him from shaving himself, tying his shoes, or fixing his meals. He is not physically able to compensate for the problem, so he is in need of assistance. Data support the nursing diagnosis "impaired physical mobility" by deduction.

Inductive reasoning

The nurse uses inductive reasoning when a patient presents with symptoms or problems the nurse has seen before. From the assessment data gathered, the nurse makes inferences (conclusions or assumptions), asks further questions, and makes decisions. The nurse, using **inductive reasoning**, goes from specifics to generalities and infers the likely outcomes based on supporting data.

For example, an RN has been working with a patient on the nursing unit for a 12-hour shift. The nurse recognizes that each time the patient is turned to the left, the blood pressure drops 15 mm Hg. The same RN has seen this phenomenon in several other patients and makes the inference that patients with right heart failure (the medical diagnosis) will experience a blood pressure drop if turned to their left side. If this patient and others with the same diagnosis do indeed become hypotensive, then the nurse becomes more confident of the reasoning. However, from the data gathered, the RN cannot yet come to a certain conclusion or formulate a nursing diagnosis. The nurse may go on to use this data, however, to support a nursing diagnosis, perhaps "fluid volume deficit, relative r/t decreased right ventricular function."

The strength of the inference is based on the extent of the RN's knowledge and experience. The RN with limited experience and with developing knowledge may rely on only the proven, is less comfortable with uncertainty, and looks to others for validation of decisions. While gaining experience and expertise, though, the nurse becomes better able to use cues from the patient and the environment to make stronger and more accurate inferences.

Elements of Reasoning and Critical Thought

Richard Paul (1995) lists eight elements as the basis of critical thought: purpose, question at issue, point of view, available information, concepts, assumptions, implications or consequences, and inferences or answers to the original purpose.

Purpose

The **purpose** recognizes that all thought has an agenda or asks the question, "What are you trying to accomplish within the context of your thought process?" An assumption exists that not all aspects of a thought are fully understood until the entire process is complete. The purpose of the inquiry thus is to answer the original question.

Question at Issue

The **question at issue** defines the purpose clearly and accurately. The question is relevant to the purpose and will allow the rest of the process to follow logically.

Point of View

All thinking stems from a **point of view**. An enlightened thinker is able to interpret data and clarify meaning from several points of view—that is, to explain or illustrate how the data can be understood from multiple positions. The RN will be able to recognize that a routine treatment may seem strange and frightening from the patient's point of view. In gathering the data to support this assumption, the nurse will ask questions to better understand how the patient is responding to the demands of the treatment. If the nurse does not understand that all thought is based on particular points of view or does not try to look at the problem from varied perspectives, then nonoptimal outcomes may result. An unenlightened nurse may make erroneous assumptions that label the patient as problematic and noncompliant.

Available Information

The thought process must be based on **available information**, data that are at hand and will give a greater understanding of the problem. Gathering historical and assessment data from the patient as well as seeking all available secondary-source information will assist the critical thinker to support the plan of care and understand the potential outcomes. Information also comes from the theoretical knowledge base of the nurse.

Concepts

As the thought process develops, **concepts** will form that begin to explain the problem at hand. A concept is an idea, theory, or mental image of something that does not yet have a tangible representation. Concepts are the structural components of the thinking process, helping us understand complex ideas, events, actions, and entities, defining and shaping our thought processes. As critical thinkers, we must be aware of how our concepts are influencing our thought processes.

Assumptions

Conceptual mental images help the thinker draw assumptions about the events, objects, or actions that are taking place. An **assumption** is an educated guess, hypothesis, or stated or unstated belief that is accepted or held as a truth without proof. Often the thought process will be based on assumptions that are taken for granted or presumed to be true but not tested or proven. In critical thinking, assumptions are challenged through inquiry as to their genuineness or their being based in reality. The RN must test assumptions before they are proven. All assumptions must be checked against the available data. If an assumption cannot be verified, then it may need to be discarded.

Implications and Consequences

Implications or **consequences** are defined through outcomes. Implications or consequences can be expected or unexpected, but each must be considered. For example, an expected consequence of bathing a patient is clean, intact skin that has a greater ability to fight infection or breakdown. Another consequence of bathing may be fatigue or chilling, which could place undue stress on the patient. The implications and consequences of thoughts, actions, and interventions must be checked and understood before completing the intervention. Every action or intervention has implications or consequences. The individual engaging in critical thought must ask the question, "What are the implications of this train of thought?" or "If I continue on this path, what will be the consequences?"

Inferences

At the completion of the systematic process of critical thought, inferences are drawn. An **inference** is the conclusion that results from, or is a summary of, the process. The nurse may be confident in the decisions made if the process is completed diligently (Paul, Elder, and Bartell, 1997).

FYI 9-1 illustrates a case study and questions related to the eight elements of reasoning and critical thought.

Structure of Critical Thought

Now that the elements of critical thought have been defined, consider the structure of the thought process. Critical thought is fluid and circular. The nursing process, at first glance, may appear linear in nature. Evaluation of the plan is expected throughout the process, yet one cannot logically design nursing interventions before problems are identified. The critical thinking process assumes that questions are formed for each step of the nursing process, asked, and answered. For example, if in the process of

FYI 9-1   Using the Eight Elements of Thought

A 68-year-old male patient with type II diabetes mellitus is being admitted for evaluation of a nonhealing wound to the left foot. To plan the patient's care using the elements of thought, the nurse would ask the following questions:

- **Purpose:** What must be accomplished with this admission? What would the priority aim be? What would be the intent of any intervention?

- **Question at issue:** What problems are present? Are any problems high priority? What is already known about the problems?

- **Information:** What empirical data (evidence) is present to support the questions at issue? What previous experiences or knowledge can be drawn upon to assist in this situation?

- **Point of view:** What are the problems as identified by the patient or the patient's family? What was going on that gave rise to the problem? What is the top-priority problem from the physician's point of view? Are the identified problems compatible or in conflict with one another? How is the top-priority problem addressed once relevant points of view have been considered?

- **Concept:** What is the main intention of the plan that is developing? Does scientific foundation or theory support the concept?

- **Assumptions:** Are any assumptions not supported by the information at hand? Are developing assumptions being ignored? What has been done or is being done to validate the assumptions being formulated?

- **Implications and consequences:** If the plan is continued, what will happen? If the interventions are implemented, what are the potential consequences? How will the interventions that are delegated or are completed by the nurse affect the patient's outcome or well being?

- **Inferences:** What are the actual conclusions to the plan? Were these conclusions expected? Do the same questions have other answers to consider?

Exercise 9-2

Besides ensuring the five rights of medication administration, what questions must you ask before giving any medication?

You enter the room of your patient in order to encourage him to cough and deep-breathe. What are you trying to accomplish by this intervention?

Before delegating a bed bath to a certified nurse assistant, what questions must you ask? What must you know about the patient and the nurse assistant?

You decide that your patient may be developing pneumonia. What information might you be using to come to that conclusion?

gathering information the nurse makes certain assumptions, then the critical thinker must process these assumptions by determining their relevance to the issue at hand and whether they are based on available data, research, or theory. Complete Exercise 9-2, answering the questions related to the structure of the thought process.

Attributes of the Critical Thinker

The nurse who engages in critical thought does so on a foundation of knowledge and other specific attributes that support the process, including curiosity, diligence in the pursuit of evidence and information, rational thought, reflection, and creativity.

Curiosity

Curiosity drives the nurse to seek knowledge in regard to the situation at hand. Curiosity is the desire to understand what something is or how it works, to be compelled to explore beyond what is immediately obvious. Curiosity may also imply skepticism, or the need to challenge beliefs in search of other possible conclusions or truths. This relentless pursuit of truth is an attribute of the curious mind. To retain an open mind, to look freshly at the world—and our patients—to practice discovery every day is curiosity realized to the fullest.

Curiosity stimulates the RN to apply all "available facts, principles, and theories" as well as specific knowledge of the situation to formulate the plan of care. Not having prejudged the situation shows the nurse to be an abstract thinker, able to derive unique solutions to best address the problems of the patient.

Diligent Pursuit of Evidence and Information

A critical thinker diligently seeks relevant evidence and information as part of the process of decision making. Collaborating with experts and consulting other references while developing the plan of care are important. The critical thinker continually assesses and responds to the patient's changing condition and makes autonomous decisions as to immediate action, within the appropriate scope of practice.

Rational Thought

Another attribute of the critical thinker is **rational thought**, which is fueled by knowledge gained through study and experience. Employing rational thought helps the nurse predict likely outcomes of planned actions or interventions, thus making sound clinical decisions based on all available information.

Reflection

To become comfortable with the process of thinking critically, the critical thinker should practice **reflection**, looking back and reconsidering ideas, thoughts, beliefs, and actions. The nurse evaluates not only the plan of care and the patient's response to nursing and medical interventions but also his or her own thought process. Reflection helps the nurse improve practice through careful self-critique of prior scenarios. In reflecting, the nurse asks whether he or she has been prejudicial or rational, considerate of other points of view or single minded, focused in the inquiry or distracted, and flexible or rigid in the thought process.

Creativity

An important attribute of the critical thinker is **creativity**, the ability to be innovative, resourceful, and inventive. Paul (1995) presents the argument that creative thinkers use critical thinking, and critical thinkers must use creative thinking principles. Creative thinking is linked to inductive reasoning in that creative thinkers recognize patterns that are present but understand that outcomes are often uncertain until tested. Each new idea generated by the creative thinker increases the number of potential outcomes to consider. If ideas are limited to those that are already accepted, then the possibilities are limited as well. Unique solutions to ambiguous problems can be found when the nurse begins by thinking creatively.

Intuitive Thought

Intuitive thought, often linked to critical thinking, involves one's sixth sense, instincts, or insight. Intuition implies perceptiveness, the ability to see or sense subtle patterns or characteristics. The intuitive nurse synthesizes data gathered from all senses and interprets the data based on past experience. Some nurses refer to this as their "gut feeling." This ability to organize minimal or vague data in order to come to conclusions is observed in the nurse who is considered an expert.

Complete Exercise 9-3, answering the questions related to the attributes of the critical thinker.

$Exercise$ 9-3

Describe a typical day as an LPN within the unit where you work:

Identify techniques you have learned to organize your day, to prioritize the tasks you must accomplish, and to make sure you have administered medication to your patients safely:

In the previous item, describe where you now see elements of critical thinking or where the inclusion of an element of critical thinking would make a positive difference in your practice:

FYI 9-2 **The Nurse as a Critical Thinker**

- Practical nursing education helps the nurse recognize important, pertinent data collected and the need to convey this information to the appropriate individual.

- The nurse who thinks critically has several attributes: curiosity, rationality, reflection, independence, creativity, fair-mindedness, and focused thinking.

- The nurse who uses critical thinking attributes to their fullest will facilitate optimal patient outcomes.

Fostering Critical Thought

Much as critical thinkers are described as having multiple attributes, the process of critical thinking is similarly multidimensional and nonlinear. With this in mind, Paul (1995) believes that the process of critical thought is rooted in discipline, which is exemplified by being true to the standards of thought and testing one's thought process for clarity, accuracy, specificity, relevance, logic, consistency, depth, and significance (FYI 9-2).

Hansten and Washburn (1999) believe it is the individual RN's responsibility to develop critical thinking skills. The process of acquiring these skills includes being open minded, valuing intuition, having the ability to self-examine and challenge one's own thought process, and having the courage to take a stand even if it is unpopular or involves a change. Furthermore, to foster critical thinking in employees, organizations must adopt a culture that accepts and encourages.

Summary

Critical thinking is a skill the RN must understand and incorporate into practice. The purpose of critical thinking is to ensure that the decision-making process will lead to the best possible patient outcomes. Critical thinking opportunities are embedded throughout the nursing process, and taking advantage of them will improve nursing care. To realize success in both personal and professional life, the nurse must consistently practice the process of critical thinking.

Critical Thinking Questions

1. From a clinical experience as a student or as an LPN, describe a situation that you feel could have been solved in a better way if sound reasoning had been used instead of emotions or feelings. How might the situation have been different, in relationship to outcomes, if rational thought had been used?

2. In response to a call light, you enter a room to find a 68-year-old patient on the floor next to the bed. The patient is in his first day post-op, surgical resection of the colon, had slept all night without complaint, and the report states that the patient had not been agitated or confused but doing well.

   a. What assumptions, if any, can you make about this situation?

   b. What are the questions that you need to ask?

References

Boychuk Duchscher JE: Catching the wave: understanding the concept of critical thinking, *J Adv Nurs* 29(3):577, 1999.

Chase SK: The social context of critical care clinical judgment, *Heart Lung* 24(2):154, 1995.

Gordon JM: Congruency on defining critical thinking by nurse educators and non-nurse scholars, *J Nurs Educ* 39(8):340, 2000.

Greenwood J: Critical thinking and nursing scripts: the case for the development of both, *J Adv Nurs* 31(2):428, 2000.

Hansten RI, Washburn MJ: Individual and organizational accountability for development of critical thinking, *J Nurs Adm* 29(11):39, 1999.

Paul R: *Critical thinking: how to prepare students for a rapidly changing world,* Santa Rosa, Cal, 1995, Foundation for Critical Thinking.

Paul R, Elder L, Bartell T: *California teacher preparation for instruction in critical thinking: research findings and policy recommendations,* Sacramento, 1997, Commission of Teacher Credentialing.

Chapter 10

Knowledge and Skill Acquisition

Key Terms

accountability
caring
chain of command
competent nurse
expert nurse
mentor
novice nurse
occurrence report

patient care
  management
proficient nurse
quality of care
root-cause analysis
standards of care
standards of practice

Overview

Your studies are preparing you to become a registered nurse. At the completion of your RN educational program, you are expected to be capable of safely managing the care of a variety of patients. Knowledge and skill acquisition is a lifelong endeavor providing growth.

This chapter assists the student in transition from LPN to RN to recognize his or her role in the continuation of knowledge and skill acquisition. We investigate personal and professional accountability in relationship to nurse practice acts, professional practice standards, and standards of care; recruiting help; and assessing outcomes through quality of care issues. These topics are explored in relationship to the RN's role in maintaining educational competency. This chapter also helps the student understand where he or she will be upon graduation, how to continue acquiring knowledge and experience in order to advance in nursing, ways to maintain accountability for professional and personal development, and how to maintain personal motivation and self-esteem (FYI 10-1).

Classification of Nursing Skill

Benner (1984) suggests that the graduate nurse enters the workforce as an advanced beginner. Del Bueno (2000) believes that the expectation for the novice RN is safe practice within set performance standards. While

---

FYI 10-1   RN Success Tools

In order to succeed as a nurse, you must provide the tools needed to do the following:

- Become a registered nurse who will advance yourself as well as the profession

- Be accountable to yourself and the profession within the nursing role

- Maintain self-esteem and motivation as a means to becoming an expert nurse

acquiring experience and skills as well as continuing with learning, the nurse will advance in a predictable pattern toward becoming an expert nurse (Benner 1984; Benner, Tanner, and Chesla, 1997; Del Bueno 2000). Specific characteristics distinguish the novice, competent, proficient, and expert nurses, and each type of nurse makes decisions and gives care in specific ways.

A **novice nurse** is a beginner, having beginning skills and lacking experience. Generally, a novice is rule driven, is a concrete thinker, and believes and trusts whomever has authority or whatever direction is perceived to have come from someone in authority. A **competent nurse** has some experience and has developed safe organizational skills to get through the day's tasks efficiently. Flexibility within the nursing role is difficult to manage at this point, and when deviations from the schedule occur, the nurse generally has a feeling of unease. A **proficient nurse** has much experience and a beginning ability to recognize patterns and think critically. The proficient nurse is able to adapt to change and might have garnered the admiration and respect of peers. An **expert nurse** has had a great deal of experience and is flexible and adaptable, responding to change with ease. The expert nurse is a skilled critical thinker.

Performance and Experience

Performance evaluations are designed to distinguish the RN's performance as being at either the novice/safe level, the competent level, or an expert level (Del Bueno, 2000). The RN gains expertise through experience and knowledge and improved critical thinking abilities. Additionally, while gaining experience, the RN begins to think more broadly and deeply. The RN also begins to acknowledge his or her investment in the human experiences of the patient, which allows more caring inquiry, enabling the RN to make more accurate clinical judgments. The expert RN can recognize minute changes in patient conditions that will assist in planning precisely individualized care (Benner, Tanner, and Chesla, 1996). A minimal expectation of the RN would be the striving for excellence and the maintenance of skill and knowledge currency while continuing professional growth. Among the major concepts later discussed within this chapter are personal and professional accountability. Subconcepts to be identified include caring, quality of care, and personal self-improvement.

Professional Accountability

Accountability is being answerable for the actions or interventions one performs as a nurse. Accountability also means taking responsibility for one's other actions and growth. Although individuals are ultimately accountable to themselves, the RN is particularly accountable to the patient, society, and the profession.

The nurse has been given professional capacity through licensure and by the job description. Standards of practice and standards of care are set by the profession as the benchmarks for judging nursing care. Individual state boards of nursing define the scope of practice and licensure requirements for RNs and LPNs, or the **standards of practice**. Each state establishes a nurse practice act, which sets legal boundaries for nursing. Boards of nursing have jurisdiction over RN and LPN licenses and decide on legal action to be taken against them. State and national nursing organizations and specialty organizations establish policies and provide position statements defining **standards of care** for nurses. Held to high standards of practice and care, the RN must know and understand both the state practice acts and the position statements on practice standards.

Quality of Care

Caring is an attribute the nurse displays through compassionate support of the patient. The caring RN is considerate of the patient's needs and reflects on how the plan of care may have a positive influence on patient outcomes. The caring RN must strive for excellence as a means to maintain **quality of care**, which is a measure of patient satisfaction and of outcomes as means for rating the attributes of patient care. Patients should be cared for in the best possible manner by compassionate nurses who demonstrate competency and proficiency. The RN who strives for a high level of expertise by following standards of practice in a caring way will maintain a high level of quality of care.

Patient Care Management

The RN is in charge of **patient care management**, which is the development of a plan of care based on assessed patient responses to medical interventions and the illness state of the patient. This includes the coordination, implementation, and evaluation of the plan. Crucial to the management of patient care are the elements of prioritization, delegation, and collaboration. One of the realities the nurse faces after graduation is not knowing everything necessary to manage the patients. End-of-the-day frustrations sometimes leave the beginning RN wondering why he or she entered nursing in the first place.

Educational and Professional Standards

Perhaps your educational goal was to gain more knowledge and experience. You attended an institution that had predetermined basic requirements for graduation, its educational standards established by schools of nursing, state boards of nursing, the National League for Nursing (NLN) Accrediting Commission, and other professional nursing organizations. Graduates are qualified to sit for the NCLEX-RN examination by meeting a minimum standard set forth by the state-accredited school of nursing and should be able to meet state and national standards for safe practice.

A large measure of trust is placed on each graduate because no single exam or course of study can predict how well or how safely an individual will actually practice. Practice policies and standards establish limits and benchmark the graduate's ability to give safe and effective care, but professional accountability and the burden of proof for one's individual competence falls to the graduate. This can be an overwhelming feeling for the graduate beginning to work in the new RN role. One of the ways to cope with the new role and responsibilities is to commit to a period of intensive learning. Personal accountability for this learning will go a long way to help the newly graduated RN cope with this change.

Personal Accountability

The individual RN should maintain a current level of expertise. Nurse practice acts mandate specific individual RN responsibilities related to continued education and competency updates. State boards of nursing may maintain specific requirements of continuing educational units. Professional standards of care as defined by peers through professional organizations, such as the National League for Nursing and the American Nurses Association (ANA), outline expected levels of expertise and experience for clinical areas.

In some states failing to maintain currency through continuing education may result in the inability to renew the RN license. Although it benefits an institution for staff LPNs and RNs to have current experience and expertise, the institution will not necessarily meet all of a nurse's continuing education needs. Unit-specific orientation with formal courses may be provided by the institution, and additional unit-specific updates are often offered regarding procedural or equipment changes or treatment plans. The scope of RN practice is much broader than these courses, however, and the RN must seek other means to remain current.

The new graduate must make an honest assessment of weaknesses and strengths related to the chosen work area. Write out your personal and professional goals, as well as steps toward accomplishment of those goals, and place them where you will see them daily. The new RN needs to schedule monthly evaluations with the supervisor to determine how well the goals are being met. The RN who uses this or a similarly proactive approach to development is assuming both professional and personal accountability. See FYI 10-2 for highlights of accountablity in registered nursing.

Professional Practice Standards and Standards of Care

Professional nursing organizations—such as the ANA, NLN, and Critical Care Nurses Association—and other specialty organizations set policies and practice standards (see FYI 10-3 for a list of professional nursing organizations). The ANA Code for Nurses defines the fundamental ethical standard under which the nurse will practice. In ethical and professional actions, the registered nurse is expected to act fairly, judicially, and professionally. The RN's judgment must be based on continuous acquisition of knowledge. The code also requires the RN to provide

Text continued on page 173

FYI 10-2 Accountability in Registered Nursing

1. The RN is accountable to self, patients, and the profession of nursing.

2. Practice standards, policies, and state nurse practice acts define limits as well as the scope of the RN's role.

3. Patients deserve quality, caring, compassionate nursing.

4. An RN who strives for excellence will gain greater trust from patients.

FYI 10-3   Partial List of Professional Nursing Organizations

Academy of Medical-Surgical Nurses

E. Holly Ave, Box 56
Pitman, NJ 08071-0006
Phone 609-256-2323, Fax 609-589-7463
E-mail: amsn@mail.ajj.com
Website: amsn.inurse.com

American Academy of Nurse Practitioners

Capitol Station, LBJ Building
PO Box 12846
Austin, TX 78711
Phone 512-442-4262, Fax 512-442-5221
E-mail: admin@aanp.org
Website: www.aanp.org

American Academy of Nursing

600 Maryland Ave, SW, Suite 100 West
Washington, DC 20024-2571
Phone 202-651-7238, Fax 202-544-2641
E-mail: lzeck@ana.org
Website: www.nursingworld.org/aan

American Assembly for Men in Nursing

c/o NYSNA
11 Cornell Rd
Latham, NY 12110-1499
Phone 518-782-9400, ext. 346, Fax 518-782-9530
E-mail: aamn@aamn.org
Website: www.aamn.org

American Association of Critical-Care Nurses

101 Columbia
Alisa Viejo, CA 92656-1491
Phone 800-899-2226, Fax 714-362-2020

Continued

E-mail: info@aacn.org
Website: www.aacn.org

American Association of Diabetes Educators

100 W. Monroe St, 4th Floor
Chicago, IL 60603
Phone 312-424-2426, Fax 312-424-2427
E-mail: styler@aadenet.org
Website: www.aadenet.org

American Association of Legal Nurse Consultants

4700 W. Lake Ave
Glenview, IL 60025-1485
Phone 847-375-4713, Fax 847-375-4777
E-mail: info@aalnc.org
Website: www.aalnc.org

American Association of Nurse Anesthetists

222 S. Prospect Ave
Park Ridge, IL 60068-4001
Phone 847-692-7050, Fax 847-692-6968
E-mail: info@aana.com
Website: www.aana.com

American Association of Occupational Health Nurses, Inc.

2920 Brandywine Rd, Suite 100
Atlanta, GA 30341
Phone 770-455-7757, Fax 770-455-7271
E-mail: aaohn@aaohn.org
Website: www.aaohn.org

American College of Nurse Practitioners

503 Capitol Ct, NE, #300
Washington, DC 20002
Phone 202-546-4825, Fax 202-546-4797
E-mail: acnp@nurse.org
Website: www.nurse.org/acnp

American Holistic Nurses Association

PO Box 2130
Flagstaff, AZ 86003-2130
Phone 800-278-2462, Fax 520-526-2752
E-mail: ahna-flag@flaglink.com
Website: www.ahna.org

American Nurses Association

600 Maryland Ave, SW, Suite 100 West
Washington, DC 20024
Phone 800-274-4262, Fax 202-554-2262
Website: www.nursingworld.org

American Psychiatric Nurses Association

1200 19th St, NW, Suite 300
Washington, DC 20036-2422
Phone 202-857-1133, Fax 202-223-4579
E-mail: apna@dc.sba.com
Website: www.apna.org

American Society of Pain Management Nurses

7794 Grow Dr
Pensacola, FL 32514
Phone 888-342-7766, Fax 850-484-8762
E-mail: aspmn@aol.com

Association of Nurses in AIDS Care

11250 Roger Bacon Dr, Suite 8
Reston, VA 20190-5202
Phone 800-260-6780, Fax 703-435-4390
E-mail: aidsnurses@aol.com
Website: www.podi.com/aids

Association of Operating Room Nurses, Inc.

2170 S Parker Rd, Suite 300
Denver, CO 80231-5711
Phone 800-755-2676, Fax 303-750-3212
Website: www.aorn.org

Continued

Association of Pediatric Oncology Nurses

4700 W Lake Ave
Glenview, IL 60025
Phone 847-375-4724, Fax 847-375-4777
E-mail: apon@amtec.com
Website: www.apon.org

Association of Rehabilitation Nurses

4700 W Lake Ave
Glenview, IL 60025-1485
Phone 800-229-7530, Fax 847-375-4777
E-mail: info@rehabnurse.org
Website: www.rehabnurse.org

Intravenous Nurses Society

10 Fawcett St
Cambridge, MA 02138
Phone 617-441-3008, Fax 617-441-3009
E-mail: ins@ins1.org
Website: www.ins1.org

National Association of Hispanic Nurses

1501 16th St, NW
Washington, DC 20036
Phone 202-387-2477, Fax 202-483-7183
E-mail: nahn@juno.com
Website: www.incacorp.com/nahn

National Association of Neonatal Nurses

1304 Southpoint Blvd, Suite 280
Petaluma, CA 94954-6861
Phone 800-451-3795, Fax 707-762-0401
E-mail: nannmbrs@aol.com
Website: www.nann.org

National Association of Orthopaedic Nurses, Inc.

E Holly Ave, Box 56
Pitman, NJ 08071-0056
Phone 609-256-2310, Fax 609-589-7463

E-mail: naon@mail.ajj.com
Website: naon.inurse.com

National Association of Pediatric Nurse Associates and Practitioners

1101 Kings Hwy North, Suite 206
Cherry Hill, NJ 08034-1912
Phone 609-667-1773, Fax 609-667-7187
E-mail: info@napnap.org
Website: www.napnap.org

National Black Nurses Association, Inc.

1511 K St, NW, Suite 415
Washington, DC 20005
Phone 202-393-6870, Fax 202-347-3808
E-mail: nbna@erols.com
Website: www.nbna.org

National Council of State Boards of Nursing, Inc.

676 N St. Clair St, Suite 550
Chicago, IL 60611-2921
Phone 312-787-6555, Fax 312-787-6898
Website: www.ncsbn.org

National Federation of Licensed Practical Nurses, Inc.

1418 Aversboro Rd
Garner, NC 27529-4547
Phone 800-948-2511, Fax 919-779-5642
E-mail: cbarbour@ntwrks.com
Website: www.nflpn.com

National Gerontological Nursing Association

7250 Parkway Dr, Suite 510
Hanover, MD 21076
Phone 800-723-0560, Fax 410-712-4424
E-mail: susan.sibiski@mosby.com

National League for Nursing

61 Broadway
New York, NY 10006

Continued

Phone 800-669-9656, Fax 613-591-4240
E-mail: nlnweb@nln.org
Website: www.nln.org

National Student Nurses Association

555 W 57th St
New York, NY 10019
Phone 212-581-2211, Fax 212-581-2368
E-mail: nsna@nsna.org
Website: www.nsna.org

Oncology Nursing Society

501 Holiday Dr
Pittsburgh, PA 15220-2749
Phone 412-921-7373, Fax 412-921-6565
E-mail: member@ons.org
Website: www.ons.org

Respiratory Nursing Society

7794 Grow Dr
Pensacola, FL 32514
Phone 888-330-4767, Fax 850-484-8762
E-mail: rnsat@aol.com

Society of Vascular Nursing

7794 Grow Dr
Pensacola, FL 32514
Phone 888-536-4786, Fax 850-484-8762
E-mail: svnatpns@aol.com

Wound, Ostomy and Continence Nurses Society

1550 S Coast Hwy, #201
Laguna Beach, CA 92651
Phone 888-224-9626, Fax 949-376-3456
E-mail: coleen@adlerdrozinc.com
Website: www.wocn.org

Adapted from Wolf P: Guide to nursing organizations, *Nursing* 28(12):53, 1998.

quality care in a collaborative effort with other health care team members to meet the needs of the patient.

The ANA has also established a policy statement regarding the need for the RN to use the nursing process when developing plans of care. The assumption is that the RN works in collaboration with the physician and other health care professionals to establish plans of care. As an independent care practitioner, the RN must use knowledge, skills, and experience to make decisions. The autonomy of RNs is thus a practice standard.

The RN is responsible for meeting the needs of the patient. The decisions the RN makes will be judged against the practice standard and may have legal and ethical implications. Practice standards determine ideals, identifying what the prudent RN should do within the role. The RN's decisions will be judged against the decisions made by another RN in a similar situation. Just as RNs are judged against their peers, of equal importance is that the consumer of health care, the patient, evaluate the quality of care given. Quality of care assumes the need for patient satisfaction, for without patients, nurses would not be needed. Complete Exercise 10-1, answering the questions related to quality and priority of care.

Accountability must be the practice standard, and clinical judgment must demonstrate that the nurse is willing to be accountable. If inadequate or inaccurate data are being gathered by nurses, then the quality of care suffers and patient days and health costs increase. In the scenario in Exercise 10-1, clinical judgment regarding the needed level of care will be faulty if the standards are not being followed. Additionally, how will quality of care be addressed if the RN is negligent in adhering to basic practice standards and agency policy? The RN is in an ideal position to increase quality of care and reduce costs if acting responsibly and accepting accountability for establishing and maintaining the plan of care. This includes the need to adhere to the policies of the unit and agency to ensure that all data are available to make decisions regarding the plan of care.

The need to be accountable for every action may seem overwhelming to the beginning RN. As an RN, you will need to make independent decisions regarding the plan of care and implementing interventions. This freedom can be a powerful tool if acted upon judiciously, but accountability cannot happen in a vacuum. The RN must collaborate with all members of the health care team and elicit their expertise and cooperation.

Exercise 10-1

In a one-on-one clinical session, an instructor questions an LPN transition student with regard to the priority of care. The student is unsure as to why the patient is still on a monitored floor and is sent to investigate. Upon return, the student explains that just 2 days ago the patient was in pulmonary edema from fluid volume overload, and with the change in medications the patient received, the doctors required that the patient be closely monitored to ensure that the pulmonary edema did not recur. The instructor then asks what the patient's intake and output has been for the last 24 hours and what the patient's weight has been. The student reports that the patient has not been saving the urine for the nurses to measure and the weight check was not done this morning.

Identify the outcome priority.

What areas of accountability are in question in this situation?

Identify the standard of practice and determine whether it has been breached:

How does the outcome of this situation affect cost?

What are your responsibilities as an RN?

Each team member has something to offer to the team. Accountability also means that a team effort exists and the RN is frequently the team leader when decisions affecting the care of the patient must be made.

Managing Care Aberrances

A health team member may defer or avoid asking for assistance from a supervisor to resolve a problem or to report an error, for fear it will hurt his or her professional reputation. One may feel that going to the supervisor will set up a confrontational situation where the only resolution to the problem or mistake will be disciplinary action. The nurse may feel powerless to request help.

The RN must act judiciously and prudently in the delivery of care. By not going to the supervisor when a mistake is made and failing to demonstrate accountability for contributing to the mistake, the RN risks not only harm to the patient but also potential legal and ethical consequences. The RN needs to take a proactive approach with administration so that issues of accountability will not be so difficult to resolve.

Occurrence Reports

Errors occur every day, even in the best of health care situations. The RN directly involved in the error or who discovers the error completes the **occurrence report** to document errors in omission or commission and to document measures taken to safeguard the patient. The occurrence report for nursing error is mandated by hospital policy and is a part of quality assurance practice standards. Areas of weakness can be identified through patterns seen in these occurrence reports. A plan can then be designed that decreases errors.

Root-Cause Analysis

Root-cause analysis of an occurrence identifies the underlying causes. Root-cause analysis is designed to seek errors of process, rather than lay blame on individuals or groups. Most errors result from one or more breaks in a chain of events.

One example would be where a nurse gives the wrong medication to a patient. In a root-cause analysis, a committee is formed, which would include in this case a facilitator (usually the risk manager or performance improvement director), the nurse or nurses involved, a pharmacist, the physician, and the team leader or supervisor. The purpose of the committee is to reconstruct the events leading up to the error. By looking at the process, the committee may discover that the physician's order was unclear, that two drugs with similar names were placed next to each other in the medication-dispensing unit, or that the units of measure for the drug was unclear. Even though the process of dispensing medications is typically safeguarded with redundant checks and balances, nurses are the last check against a medication error.

Acute health care hospitals that use the root-cause analysis process generally identify solutions more accurately than hospitals that do not. These solutions include further individual or staff education, correction of a policy or procedure, or, if needed, discipline. By not making negative consequences, such as discipline, the main focus of correcting systemic or procedural problems, greater reporting of errors or problems will hopefully occur. Whether it is an individual, communication, system, or procedural problem, occurrence reporting provides a way to track and identify problem areas, which can ensure better outcomes when put through the analysis process.

The nurse must view an occurrence report as a positive step toward improving care. Quality care will not happen without evaluation. The report can identify staffing inadequacies or disparities as well as educational or training needs. Positive change cannot happen without understanding the need for change and the needs to *be* changed. A dialogue between staff nurses and unit management should be initiated to ensure that occurrence reports are used in a positive way. Unless gross negligence, assault or battery, or another felony has occurred, the occurrence report should not be used in a punitive way. Individual problems can be handled with greater supervision, education, or training, and through a specific plan that will help the individual achieve a higher level of function. Unit-specific problems may require education, increased staff support, or a greater supervisory role. All care providers, licensed and nonlicensed personnel, must be held accountable for their actions, and occurrence reporting is a means to establish accountability.

Involving Management in Decision Making

Accountability also extends to times when the nurse must involve supervisors, department managers, or the nursing or hospital administrators in the decision-making process. The RN must recognize those times when management is needed to facilitate care or to assist in operational decisions affecting care given on a unit. The staff RN is often reluctant to call unit managers, house supervisors, or administration when bed availability issues arise, for example. This includes times when the RN is required to find beds in another unit or even in another facility. While these tasks may be within the RN's collaborative role, the RN should also know when this task should be delegated to those who do not have direct patient care duties, such as the unit or house supervisor or the bed-utilization nurse. If the problem will take the RN more than a phone call to resolve, it would be taking time and energy away from patient care.

Patient and Family Complaints

Patient and family complaints are another area in which the RN may not have the experience, time, and information to intervene appropriately. The RN must determine when he or she should handle a problem personally or refer it to another appropriate resource. Resolution or not, the outcome will be dependent on the perception of the patient or family and how well the patient or family perceives that needs are being met. The RN must understand the experience, responsibilities, and accountability of different health care team members when it comes to accessing them. The RN must be prepared to resolve certain patient problems through a phone call to the unit manager or house supervisor. Pastoral care services or social services may be able to assist with other problems.

Chain of Command

The RN may be reluctant to use the chain of command when a need arises to correct a problem that threatens patient care. Each health care system has an established **chain of command**, including individuals with defined management responsibilities, from the board of directors, to health care administrator or chief operating officer, through the various levels of management, down to the nursing staff. The nurse resolves problems by beginning with the immediate supervisor, if necessary working up the chain of command to higher levels of authority. If the RN knows how to use the chain of command effectively, most problems can be resolved without a compromise to patient care. For the nurses the final step most often occurs at the director of nursing level, but the process could continue to the board of directors, if necessary.

Difficulties with communication between a physician and a nurse may lead to conflicts that compromise the standard of care. The RN must remember that not going up the chain of command in an attempt to resolve the conflict makes him or her accountable if patient care continues to be compromised.

Failing to gain cooperation from the other health care team members may make the RN's load much heavier than necessary. Input from the supervisory level can often facilitate accomplishing actions in a more timely fashion. Consistently using the appropriate chain of command reinforces the team effort to uphold the standard of patient care. The RN is accountable for the care given, and the care must be given in a judicious manner.

Quality of Care Measurement

Quality of care measurement tools gauge patient satisfaction, cost of care, and effectiveness of care. The RN, as the coordinator of care, is directly accountable for these issues. Generally, quality of care is measured through patient satisfaction surveys, chart reviews, and studies that look at specific aspects of care. Patient satisfaction has a direct influence on the revenue that the hospital receives because patient satisfaction drives the patient's decision to use the health care facility again. Therefore the RN must pay attention to quality care ratings given to health care facilities, as well as to units within these facilities.

More importantly, when an individual patient is unhappy and behaving in a negative manner, the RN must investigate this behavior and determine its source. Often it is related to pain, angst, sorrow, or anxiety. Once the source of the behavior is identified, the RN must attempt to resolve the problem with good communication and management techniques. Not surprisingly, patients are more satisfied with care that has the elements of "caring"—listening, empathy, and understanding—than when care is given in a detached and uncaring manner.

Developing Professional Relationships

The nurse must be aware of his or her personal satisfaction level with the new roles as RN. Maintaining personal integrity and motivation will be a challenge for the former LPN. When the reality of the added responsibilities becomes clear, the newly graduated RN will find ego and self-esteem challenged. Developing professional and personal relationships will assist in maintaining a sense of self. Personal relationships will be difficult if the individual focuses on only what can be gained from the relationship. Learning to give and take will take practice.

Typically, the new nurse looks to peers for assistance in making decisions. The practice of deferring decisions to a more experienced nurse is one way the new graduate can cope with overwhelming feelings. Deferring decisions will work if the graduate also learns from the expert nurse the critical thinking skills needed in order to develop confidence. Chapter 9 discusses the critical thinking tools needed to become an expert nurse; the rest of this chapter details the survival skills the RN needs for the first year of practice, plus ways to continue toward excellence.

Mentorship

The graduate RN will need to identify a **mentor**. The mentor relationship is traditionally between an established practitioner and a novice. The mentor is considered to be a wise sage who takes a new employee and teaches survival skills. The mentor assists the new employee in understanding the political and power structure of the agency. The mentor functions as a support person, coming with assistance when needed, giving advice, and sharing knowledge and experience. The newly graduated RN will use the mentor to find his or her way within the new RN role and within the health care institution.

Mentor Characteristics

The RN mentor is most likely highly proficient or considered an expert in his or her area of practice and has a desire to share knowledge. Team members look to the proficient nurse for leadership demonstrated in a cooperative style, leading by example and delegating to the expertise of the individual team members. FYI 10-4 lists some such characteristics of a mentor.

The mentor will expect the beginning RN to be an active participant in personal development, as well as to be prepared to care for the patients. Cultivation of the mentor relationship will be easier if the expert RN recognizes the effort that the beginning RN makes.

Fostering the Mentor Relationship

Effective mentors are willing to share knowledge and model high levels of thinking. The beginning nurse should emulate the thinking process of the more expert nurse, thereby gaining more confidence while gaining more

FYI 10-4   Characteristics of a Mentor

A mentor is:

1. **Trustworthy.** The mentor is supportive and sage with critique.

2. **Knowledgeable.** The mentor has skill proficiency, wisdom, and expertise.

3. **Collegial.** The mentor is respected, is willing to collaborate, and shares expertise.

4. **Politically aware.** The mentor knows how to get things accomplished, internalizes the mission of nursing, and respects the institutional mission.

5. **A skilled communicator.** The mentor is precise and thoughtful in all forms of communication.

6. **Empowering.** The mentor encourages those who put forth effort, respects those who strive for excellence, and champions their achievements.

knowledge and critical thinking ability. The best way for the beginner to access the expertise of the mentor is through sound questioning, which seeks clarification and insight into the mentor's thought process. An individual who develops a highly skilled questioning ability will learn more and be able to reason at a higher level.

The following are examples of two different approaches to solicit more information about catheters.

- Nurse number one: "What is a pulmonary catheter?"

- Nurse number two: "I read last night that with the pulmonary catheter you can determine the patient's cardiac output, pulmonary wedge pressure, and cardiac index. I think I have an idea of how it will help in making a decision about dopamine dosage, but I'm not sure exactly how to decide. Can you tell me how you decide?"

The second nurse asks a higher-level question and demonstrates preparedness. The beginning nurse who uses higher-level questioning gains more for the effort.

FYI 10-5 lists characteristics of the new RN that will assist in establishing a mentor relationship. The graduate RN should remain flexible, be willing to adjust to the learning environment, and take advantage of new experiences. By being assertive and making learning needs known, the new graduate can seek learning experiences that complement independent research. Additionally, seeking constructive input from the mentor will help the new graduate define strengths as well as areas for further learning.

Understanding the Challenges Ahead

The change process involves challenges. The LPN entering as a transition student has from 1 to several years' experience as a nurse. The LPN has had a chance to become a proficient nurse at that level and is now faced with the knowledge that he or she has much to learn before becoming proficient at the RN level. The choice to return to school, with all of its challenges, is admirable, yet to maintain motivation beyond the security of school will be an even greater challenge.

Success and Failure

Success and failure are opposite concepts. If we see the world only in terms of success and failure, however, we have missed many learning

FYI 10-5   Characteristics of an RN in a Successful Mentor Relationship

Assisting in strengthening a mentor relationship, the graduate RN is:

1. **Available for learning experiences.** The graduate RN makes his or her learning needs known, is prepared to take on new learning experiences, and is thoughtful about the learning that is taking place.

2. **Self-reliant.** The graduate RN is confident enough to ask questions, seek clarification, and seek constructive input.

3. **Respectful of the mentor's knowledge and skill.** The graduate RN understands the experience needed to gain expertise and will open a dialogue with the mentor.

4. **A strong communicator.** The graduate RN is clear, precise, and thoughtful in the questions asked and in the dialogue that follows.

5. **Empowered.** The graduate RN is hungry for learning experiences, demonstrates this through a sound plan, and is focused on the matters at hand.

opportunities, which are in every event in which we participate. Individuals who take the opportunity to learn in the face of a difficult situation can turn a potential failure into a success. Looking at a situation in a new way is called *reframing* the situation and is a positive technique that will assist in building self-confidence.

Maintaining Positive Self-Esteem

Mistakes can cause us, as caregivers, to feel bad about ourselves rather than feel bad about the mistakes. This feeling can lead us to become frustrated and can perhaps cause low self-esteem. RNs must take care to not make mistakes in the first place and to assess the reason for any errors that do occur so that they will not be repeated. There is no excuse to ignore a mistake, which could be seen as negligence. Not to learn from the mistake is also neglecting an opportunity to grow. Continual growth is essential in registered nursing.

Getting involved in institutional activities can increase the RN's sense of belonging. Volunteering for committee work and assisting in quality care surveys and community-based activities offer new nurses opportunities to establish additional professional relationships, which can lead to further advancement within the institution as well as building personal support.

RNs need to develop outside interests as well. Looking forward to activities that you enjoy at work can be a great feeling, but it can be a disappointment if you have nothing to look forward to when you leave work. Creative activities are not only valuable in developing critical thinking skills but also as ways to release energy after a difficult day of work. Exercise and sports activities promote health and relieve stress.

Additionally, family activities should not be ignored. Strong family ties and close friendships can be important support systems and a way to build self-esteem. Loved ones are more likely to build egos and act to build up self-esteem when the RN has been facing challenges in the new roles. Self-esteem and self-improvement go hand in hand. While growing stronger in skill and knowledge, you also grow stronger in confidence, which will be reflected in your work.

Summary

As a student, you are being prepared to become an RN. Accountability, quality care, and personal satisfaction are important concepts to keep in mind. The graduate nurse enters the workforce as an advanced beginner. Moving toward proficiency, the new RN acquires experience, continues learning, and gains skills, and with further progress advances to become an expert nurse.

A major concept within this chapter is personal and professional accountability. The RN is ultimately accountable to himself or herself and to the need to maintain excellence in practice. The RN is also accountable to the patient, to provide the best care possible that is safe and effective in moving the patient to a prior or higher level of function. The RN must also be accountable to the nursing profession because the profession sets practice standards, which, with standards of care, provide benchmarks for judging nursing care. Individual state boards of nursing define the scope of practice and licensure for RNs. Each state has a nurse practice act, which sets legal boundaries of nursing. A standard of practice is that RNs maintain a level of expertise for their area. As a graduate, the RN needs to seek out expert nurses and foster mentor relationships, gaining through the experience of others the necessary tools to advance. Additionally, the RN needs to recognize situations that call for assistance from managers or supervisors. Fostering positive, honest relationships with administrators will only improve patient care.

Finding ways to maintain interest in and out of the institution also assists the new RN in feeling more comfortable with the role change from LPN. Support systems are important, and the RN needs to foster them to assist with challenges.

Critical Thinking Questions

The answers to each of the following questions should use the elements of critical thinking: purpose, questions at issue, available information, basic concepts, assumptions, inferences and interpretations, implications and consequences, and point of view.

1. Identify five things about the role of the RN you believe to be important. Rank them from most important to least important to you. Get together with one other student in your class, and from your two lists, come up with three facts that you both agree upon as being most important. Then identify two other students who do not have the same, and repeat, agreeing on just three facts that the four of you believe to be most important. For each fact, answer the following questions:

   a. How would you go about supporting your assumption that these items are highly important to the role of the RN?

   b. What information would you need to prove or disprove your claim?

   c. What are the possible outcomes to not holding these to be true?

2. Your are the RN in charge. An LPN has just reported that she has just hung the O negative blood on Mr. Smith. The blood had been ordered, but you were unaware that the type and cross-match had been completed and the blood was ready.

   a. What are the standards of practice for the incident, and what action must you as RN take?

   b. Write out the incident report as it should be documented as well as the nurse's notes.

3. Your patient is to receive a bolus of 4 mg of morphine sulfate IVP and has a standing PRN order for 2 to 4 mg IVP q1h. The unit-dose syringe is 10 mg per 1 ml. After giving the 4 mg bolus, you decide that, rather than waste the rest of the medication, you will place the medication in the patient's drawer to give later. A team member RN later reports giving your patient 4 mg of the morphine from the drawer stash and wasting the rest of the medication. He wants you to cosign the pharmacy sheet account for the waste.

   a. What are the professional and legal issues?

   b. What assumption can you make, and how would you go about collecting information to support the assumptions?

References

Benner P: *From novice to expert: excellence and power in clinical nursing practice*, Menlo Park, Cal, 1984, Addison-Wesley.

Benner P, Tanner CA, Chesla CA: *Expertise in nursing practice: caring, clinical judgment, and ethics*, New York, 1997, Springer.

Del Bueno DJ: *A model for competence and success.* Presentation given at Northeast Baptist Hospital, San Antonio, Tex, March 2000.

Wolf P: Guide to nursing organizations, *Nursing* 28(12):53, 1998.

Chapter 11

The RN as a Communicator

Key Terms

communication blocker

communication
facilitator

delegation

empathy

exploration phase

initiation phase

patient's story

preparation phase

termination phase

therapeutic
communication

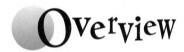Overview

Communication is an integral part of the RN role. The exchange and recording of essential information is fundamental and must be completed with clarity and precision. Competent communication is a professional standard of practice for the registered nurse.

This chapter addresses ways to improve communication skills and provides opportunities to learn the importance of competent communication. The four phases of communication—preparation, initiation, exploration or working, and termination—are explored as they relate to the various responsibilities of the RN, as are facilitators and blockers of effective communication. Examples of how the RN uses practical communication skills in obtaining health history, conducting physical assessment, and interacting therapeutically are presented. Potential solutions to communication issues with co-workers and physicians are also included. The legal implications of documentation as well as common problems found in charting and other forms of written communication are explored.

Foundation for Communication

Oermann (1997) believes that nurse-client communication is an ongoing and ever-changing transactional process with multidimensional characteristics. Environmental and personal factors are variables in any communication process. This assumption "directs people to examine factors that affect both the nurse and the client and to determine how the continuous interchange between them will vary depending on the nature of the situation" (p. 141). The RN must consider the environment in which the communication is taking place and the physical and emotional disposition and state of mind of the patient at the time of the interaction. Folsom (1999) indicates that "the beauty and art of nursing lie in the nurse-patient relationship" (p. 80). Folsom relates that using many forms of communication, such as imagery, meditation, and therapeutic touch, is needed to meet the holistic needs of patients.

The RN communicates in many different ways. The RN is responsible for effectively gathering information from the patient regarding current health concerns. This information will be shared with physicians and other health care team members. By law the RN must accurately record the patient's responses to the condition as well as the treatment plan. This becomes a legal record, is used to measure outcomes and determine costs, and may serve to defend the care given if case litigation occurs.

The RN needs to delegate duties, collaborate with many health care departments, and confer with other health care providers in order to carry out the plan of care. As a patient advocate, the RN must be able to assist the patient in understanding his or her own health concerns. The RN must also understand when therapeutic communication is needed to assist the patient and others in coping with their concerns or problems. As a patient advocate, the RN must assist the patient toward understanding of treatment options, disease process, and prognosis.

Similar to the RN, you have already been using communication as a tool within your role as an LPN. You have been passing on and receiving information, acting as patient advocate, and using communication to comfort and care for the patient. In this role you have recognized situations when communication has both hampered and helped you.

Communication is an interaction between two or more individuals in which an exchange of information occurs. For communication to occur, an expression from one individual must be received by at least one other. A dialogue will take place, and there will be an acknowledgment of mutual understanding of the exchange. Communication can be either verbal (spoken or written) or nonverbal (body language). In general, nonverbal communication is considered to offer more "truth" than verbal communication. Therefore the nurse must be constantly aware of and managing his or her nonverbal communication (Taylor, Lillis, and LeMone, 2001).

Communication, like any skill, has elements and principles. Good communication evolves by your practicing correct principles and using the elements appropriately. Recognizing this, plan to refer to your past experiences in applying the new knowledge you will gain about communication (FYI 11-1).

Therapeutic Communication

When a nurse engages in a helping relationship with a patient and family, **therapeutic communication** is at the heart of the interaction (FYI 11-2). During the interviewing process, the patient may disclose a number of concerns. The RN should try to understand such concerns with both sensitivity and empathy. Therapeutic communication requires

FYI 11-1   Communication Fundamentals

The RN must demonstrate fundamental competency in several aspects of communication:

- Motivation to maintain competent communication is a standard of practice.

- Communication in all aspects of the RN's day must be accurate, understandable, and fair.

- RN-client communication is a process with multidimensional characteristics.

- The RN must be aware of all factors that affect communication. The time frame before the surgery, or for any procedure, is typically short, yet the standard of care requires the RN to teach the patient about the care.

- The RN's communication must have relevance and a purpose in order to establish a caring relationship with the patient.

- The RN must establish effective communication with all health care team members.

FYI 11-2   Phrases that Illustrate Therapeutic Communication

- Tell me more about . . .

- I heard you say . . .

- You sound angry [sad, hurt, anxious]; can you tell me about it?

- I understand you want [need, feel] . . .

- It must be hard for you to tell me how you are feeling.

- Sometimes when I feel sad [angry, anxious, hurt], I find myself . . . Is that how you see it as well?

empathy, being able to maintain compassionate insight into the feelings and beliefs of the individual, accept with thoughtful consideration his or her point of view, and maintain awareness of the influence of your own words, intonation, and nonverbal gestures.

Communication Facilitators

A factor that enhances effective communication is a **communication facilitator**. The nurse must project warmth, acceptance, friendliness, openness, empathy, and respect in all interactions with the patient and family. Remain patient focused to demonstrate that you care for the person, not the disease, the room number, or the bed number. Project to the patient that he or she is more than just another item on the to-do list for the shift.

Another communication facilitator is providing for the privacy, confidentiality, and comfort of the patient. In addition, be mindful of the pace of your words and actions. Appropriate humor and touch can help foster a closer nurse-patient relationship.

If your patient is experiencing an impaired ability to communicate, such as in the case of intubation, aphasia, a voice problem, dysarthria, or a hearing problem, you should find alternate means to communicate.

Patients enter the health care system under difficult situations, which often evokes powerful emotions. An angry, hurting, or grieving patient may be confrontational, passive, highly emotional, or crying uncontrollably. Even though outward demonstrations of emotions may be directed at health care workers, the actual emotions may be a result of the patient's perception of how the health care concerns are affecting his or her life. In a situation where a patient is directing anger at the RN or other health care workers, your maintaining silence, nodding in acknowledgment of the anger, and seeking clarification through careful questioning can bring about understanding of the reason behind the behavior. Health care workers must avoid taking patient behavior personally.

Communication Blockers

A **communication blocker** tends to stop conversation and build mistrust (FYI 11-3). The RN has many time constraints, duties, and decisions to make. These will often be on the nurse's mind when approaching a patient in distress. Condescending language can also block conversation.

FYI 11-3   **Examples of Blockers and Facilitators to Therapeutic Communication**

The following is a conversation with communication blockers:

Patient: I feel as though I can't get my breath when I walk down the street.

RN: What else makes you short of breath? *More like a detective, this RN gives a nontherapeutic response that does not acknowledge what is important to the patient. The RN who uses this type of question is generally trying to get through with the interviewing process.*

Patient: I don't know; I just can't walk very far, and I just have a hard time.

RN: Tell me what other problems you have. *Like with the response above, the RN still seems primarily interested in finishing the interview, perhaps the health history. In this case, furthermore, the RN is ignoring the patient's concern.*

Patient: Well, umm, just can't get to the corner store like I used to.

RN: Well, okay, then. I will tell your doctor what you said to me. Is there anything else I can help you with? *In this response, the RN is deflecting responsibility to solve the problem. Rather than being understanding, the RN projects an unconcerned attitude.*

The following is a conversation that facilitates trust:

Patient: I feel as though I can't get my breath when I walk down the street.

RN: You can't get your breath when you are walking outside? Is this the only time you feel you have trouble breathing? *In this response, the RN restates what the patient has said. This tells the patient that you heard him or her and allows you to probe further. It says to the patient that you want to know what he or she has to say and that you have time to listen.*

Patient: Well, no. I get short of breath whenever I walk any distance. I used to be able to go to the neighborhood store, and now I can't seem to walk to the end of my driveway before I have trouble.

RN: So walking is getting harder for you lately. It sounds as though you are concerned that you are not able to do what you used to be able to do. What are you still able to do for yourself? *Empathy, a critical component of therapeutic conversation, projects understanding of the main concern* *of the patient. Here the nurse projects empathy by focusing on the main concern.*

Patient: Oh, I am able to get my mail, let the dog in and out, and I can get around the house all right, but I sit and rest more than I used to.

Questioning a patient's reasons rather than accepting them will block therapeutic communication. "Why" questions or ones that challenge the patient, such as "What did you do that for?" or "Did you really do that?" are considered to be blockers. Try saying, "I'm having a hard time understanding; can you please clarify for me just how this happened?" Asking questions in this manner encourages the patient and family to share openly. Nonjudgmental acceptance of the information revealed is expected.

Other blocks to communication include a task-oriented approach to nursing care. The task-oriented nurse thinks of the patient in terms of what needs to be done. Referring to the patient using only a room and bed number does not convey a personal approach. Failing to listen attentively, offering unsolicited advice or false reassurances, using clichés, or engaging in gossip will all damage the nurse-patient relationship.

The RN and all health care workers should be aware of how their communication skills affect patients and patient care. Minimizing communication blockers while maximizing therapeutic interventions leads to greater patient satisfaction and positive patient outcomes. In FYI 11-4, several facilitating and blocking communication techniques are listed.

Phases of Communication

The nurse's communication with the patient and family as well as with other members of the health care team will follow basic phases and principles. The basic phases of communication are preparation, initiation, exploration, and termination. Each phase is enhanced by following basic principles, such as actively listening and showing respect for the speaker's beliefs. The following sections present these basic phases with techniques that facilitate effective communication.

FYI 11-4   Blockers and Facilitators to Therapeutic Communication

The following are blockers to therapeutic communication:

- Making irrelevant comments

- Making ambiguous comments

- Interrupting the patient

- Not responding when a response to the patient is called for

- Using too familiar or impersonal language

- Changing the subject or otherwise shifting the focus away from the patient's concerns

- Turning away from the patient or becoming distracted

- Inappropriately kidding or joking

- Displaying annoying ticks or habits, such as tapping a foot

The following are ways to facilitate therapeutic communication:

- Responding directly to the patient's statements

- Nodding one's head or leaning toward the patient

- Staying on the topic at hand or directing the topic toward the major concerns

- Showing verbal and nonverbal interest in and awareness of what is being said

- Expressing understanding of what is being said or seeking clarification toward understanding

- Elaborating on the content, giving examples in order to broaden understanding

- Presenting hypotheses or assumptions, seeking clarification for validation

Preparation Phase

In the **preparation phase**, before beginning a conversation with a patient, the RN reviews available information (FYI 11-5). Perhaps other health care team members have gathered information. Getting to know the **patient's story** begins with understanding the circumstances that led the patient to seek health care. The EMT report, the admission record, the doctor's admitting notes, available diagnostic reports, and the report from the admitting RN are some of the resources for preparing for the initial contact with the patient. Benner, Tanner, and Chesla (1996, 1997) believe that by understanding the patient's story, the expert nurse is able to recognize subtle changes in the patient's condition. Benner later (1999) states, "Nursing is concerned with the social sentient body that dwells in finite human worlds; that gets sick and recovers; that is altered during illness, pain, and suffering; and that engages with the world differently upon recovery. Concern with how the body engages and is engaged in specific local worlds is at the heart of the caring practice of nursing" (p. 315). Establishing a caring relationship with a patient requires the RN to be engaged in understanding the patient's story. To be engaged, the RN must access preliminary information about the patient as a means to begin the process of knowing the story. From this preliminary knowledge, the RN will begin to formulate a sense of the patient's concerns, making assumptions to be checked later by the questioning process.

FYI 11-5 Understanding the Patient's Story

The RN who begins the communication process prepared will have valuable information for formulating a sound understanding of the patient's story.

- In understanding the patient's story, the RN is in the best position to recognize subtle changes.

- The RN engaged in understanding the patient's story is at the "heart of the caring practice of nursing."

- The RN must plan for sufficient communication time in order to understand the patient's story.

Perhaps the RN is the first to greet the patient and there is no history available. Preparation would then begin as the RN enters the room and surveys the situation. This means the RN pays attention to the verbal and nonverbal information given by the patient and family members to assist in preparing for the interview. Posture, facial expression, and general appearance can determine the patient's readiness to be interviewed. In addition, your acknowledging and meeting needs, such as pain or anxiety, before conducting the interview may increase the patient's willingness to develop a trusting relationship.

Do not develop assumptions. Unconfirmed assumptions, or unasked questions because of improper preparation, can lead to erroneous conclusions. Without prior information you run a high risk for developing false or even prejudicial beliefs and misconceptions about the patient or situation, which may hinder developing a trusting relationship and impair your ability to deliver optimal patient care. Exercise 11-1 illustrates a scenario in which staff RNs made erroneous assumptions as a result of an incomplete patient story.

During a typical day within the health care setting, the RN will obtain the patient's health history and physical examination, continue the assessment or evaluation of the patient's needs, and inquire into problems. During such preparation phase interactions, the RN must plan sufficient time to engage in conversations and allow for the patient's story to be told as completely as possible. Generally, a practiced interview process can take as short as 20 minutes or as long as 60. To ensure adequate uninterrupted time, the RN will need to delegate other responsibilities, as appropriate, to team members. The RN may have to explain to the patient the need to break up the interview into shorter intervals intentionally rather than conduct it all at once. You must keep the patient informed of your responsibilities while assuring the patient that you will meet his or her needs. Organization is important, and a relaxed, unhurried approach is most effective to obtain the needed data.

The patient's family can be a great source of information about the patient's history. The family can relate changes that they have seen, set time frames, and introduce the spiritual, emotional, and cultural concerns of the patient. Benner, Tanner, and Chesla (1997) believe that within the patient's world, the family holds a principal position. The nurse who solicits the family for information will gain greater understanding of the patient. In addition, you will be in a position to include the family in the plan of care. The RN who is familiar with all available information gathered

Exercise 11-1

The father of a 3-year-old child hospitalized with complications of cystic fibrosis and pneumonia had been in the pediatric intensive care unit by the child's side for the first 48 hours. The last few days before the child was discharged from the unit, the father had left only to go to work, sleeping at the child's bedside each night. During the child's hospitalization, the mother had not been seen, although she had called several times. The RNs in the pediatric intensive care unit had assumed that the mother was not devoted to the child, and many of the RNs expressed anger that she had not come to visit.

The father was interviewed as part of a research project to determine the needs of family members of patients in intensive care units. During the interview process it was discovered that this family also had an older child with cystic fibrosis. The father expressed that what he needed most was the assurance that his wife was taking care of this other child. This need for internal family support had developed over the years while they coped with having children with chronic illnesses. The couple decided that one parent would stay home to care for the one child, while the other would be with the hospitalized child. In this case the mother would continue the older child's treatments at home. They reasoned that they could reduce the risk of giving this older child pneumonia if, for the duration of the younger child's illness, they gave separate care to each child, not risking carrying the pneumonia home to the older child (Corbin, 1990).

What could be the consequences of the nurses not knowing the whole story?

What questions could the nurses ask to help them understand the patient's story with more accuracy?

before entering the patient's room better understands the severity of the situation, can relate the condition to similar situations, and can better understand the specific individual nature of the patient's condition. The family, the patient's chart, and shift reports build the frame of reference for new data from which clinical judgments may be made.

Initiation Phase

The main purpose of the **initiation phase**, also known as the orientation phase, is for the development of a trusting relationship with the patient (FYI 11-6). During this phase the nurse begins to gather information directly from the patient. The nurse and patient or family members should come to know each other by name. Write your name so the patient can read it and have it at hand. Communication should be purposeful and patient focused. In the initiation phase of the communication process, the RN and patient establish a verbal agreement, or contract, that includes the purpose or need, expected time frame, boundaries and limitations, and roles and responsibilities. During this phase the nurse provides orientation to the patient regarding the facility, unit, and room, ensuring to point out devices such as the call bell and to explain any initial orders left by the physician.

Factors Influencing the Initiation Phase   Many positive and negative influences affect the establishment of a trusting relationship.

FYI 11-6   Preparing for Communication

- Establishing a nurse-patient contract facilitates a trusting relationship.

- Patient concerns are to be respected, and the RN should plan questions that are sensitive to the patient's beliefs.

- Assessing the patient's readiness and willingness to engage in communication is important to maintain positive outcomes.

- The RN must establish a therapeutic environment for effective communication to take place.

The patient must be invited and encouraged to become an active member in the nurse-patient relationship. The RN needs to understand the patient's point of view and not interject his or her own beliefs or prejudices.

SENSITIVE ISSUES Another barrier the RN must understand is that the patient's personal beliefs may have an influence on willingness or even ability to answer questions readily. Specific questions may embarrass or offend an individual. Pose questions in such a way that the importance of the information is sensitively communicated to the patient. The patient also needs to feel secure that the information will be confidential and communicated only to those with need to know. The patient may also need permission to not share information he or she is uncomfortable in disclosing. However, if the patient feels secure and the nurse has successfully established trust, then cooperation will be more forthcoming.

The barrier may not be the way a question is asked but who might be asking the question, perhaps because of gender. A male patient may have difficulty answering a female RN regarding problems with urination or erections. Equally awkward may be a female patient being asked questions by a male RN regarding problems with her breasts or reproductive organs. Perhaps such a part of the interview should be deferred to a nurse whose gender is the same as the patient's. When this accommodation is not possible, assure the patient that as a nurse, your primary concern is his or her needs and carry on in a matter-of-fact manner. Cultural or personal patient beliefs may also determine who should or should not be given intimate access to the patient.

PATIENT CONDITION The RN must also consider the patient's condition during this initiation phase. The patient may be so fatigued, weak, ill, sedated, in pain, in a state of agitation, or mentally incapable as to be unable to engage in a conversation. Before beginning a conversation, ask the patient whether he or she has any needs that should be taken care of first. Alleviating pain, allowing the patient to satisfy elimination needs, and adjusting the bed to a comfortable position will all help establish a therapeutic environment. In some cases, you should set an interview time for when the patient will feel rested or pain free.

ENVIRONMENT The initiation phase is also the time to set the environment for the conversation. As much privacy should be arranged as possible.

Ask visitors to leave, turn off the television, and eliminate all other distracting noise, and provide enough light. Eye contact is important to the interviewing process. Sit in a position so that you can be seen, preferably at eye level, and you can see the patient. Lighting is important because it allows both parties to see each other clearly and respond to nonverbal communication, such as gestures, facial expressions, and posture, which contribute to the validity of the information exchange. Eyeglasses and any hearing-assistance devices should be in place.

Both the patient and the nurse need to be comfortable. By sitting in a chair you will demonstrate that you have time to spend with the patient and that the information provided is valued. The space between you and the patient should be respectful of the patient's personal space but close enough to indicate that you are interested in what is being said. Respond to the patients' cues; watch for open gestures, such as palms up or eye contact, and closed gestures, such as arms crossed over the torso or lack of eye contact.

Exploration Phase

The **exploration phase** is the "working phase" and the longest phase, indeed the essence of the nurse-patient relationship. It begins with the nursing assessment, interview, and physical examination. Responding to patient cues, the RN develops a series of questions and completes an assessment that allows identification of patient concerns. As problems are identified, the nurse prioritizes the list and collaborates with the patient to design a plan of care. All interactions during this phase are deliberately planned, implemented, and evaluated in concert with the patient to reach the mutually specified goals. The exploration phase lasts until the agreed time frame, usually at the conclusion of the patient stay.

LISTENING   One of the most important skills an RN can master in support of this phase is the skill of listening. Listening requires clarification and verification of what the patient is saying. Use questions that seek clarification: "You told the doctor about . . . What more can you tell me?" "Clarify something you said earlier; you mentioned . . ." "You say your pain is in your chest; how would you describe the pain?" The RN should project careful listening. A strained posture, poor eye contact, or constant distracting movements or habits, such as chewing gum or jingling pocket change, would communicate disinterest in what the patient is saying.

The nurse should note questions already asked, including by others, and answered. During the admission process some questions will appear to be redundant, and a patient can become frustrated with many people asking the same or similar questions, perceiving that no one is really listening. The nursing admission form has questions that the physician or other health care professionals have already asked and documented. Reviewing the chart before conducting the interview will save time and energy for both you and the patient. Let the patient know that any redundant questions are for the purpose of verifying information already documented.

ORIENTATION OF QUESTIONS AND EXPLANATIONS   Even though medical terminology is frequently seen and heard in the media, both in news reporting and in entertainment programs, we must not assume that the patient will understand questions that include medical terms and jargon. However, it is equally important not to "talk down" to the patient. In every interaction, you must assess the patient's knowledge level, educational background, and health care experiences to determine the appropriate orientation of the explanation (FYI 11-7).

FYI 11-7   Opening Questions

- Tell me what your concerns are? *This is a broad opening question that will allow the patient to begin to share concerns. Such a broad opening statement will allow the nurse to begin at the patient's level of understanding, but following questions must be more focused.*

- I see that you told the doctor you were "not feeling well." Can you tell me more about how you are feeling? How is it different now from how you normally feel? *This type of question is useful if there is an identified chief concern, but clarification is needed. Again, followup questions will become more focused.*

- You say that you have been having "this problem" for a while now. Tell me what changed that led you to seek help for the problem at this time? *This question is helpful if you feel a patient might have delayed getting medical help. It also may be helpful to identify a readiness on the part of the patient to make a significant life change that can assist in a healthier way of living.*

A patient may misunderstand even a fairly common word, such as *allergy.* If asked about whether he or she has any allergies, the patient may simply reply with a yes or a no. Often the patient who answers no might not have considered food or environmental allergies as important or might not have understood that the reactions to foods he or she eats may be allergic reactions. At a time when a patient answers yes regarding a medication allergy, he or she might have equated medication side effects with an allergic reaction. Perhaps you should ask whether the patient has had any "problematic reactions" to medications or foods. Then the nurse can elicit more information and determine whether the reaction was an allergic response or a side effect.

Be flexible when conducting the health history. Determining the chief complaint helps you determine the order in which to collect the rest of the health history data. Questions such as "What were you doing just before deciding to seek help?" and "What do you think caused you to feel this way?" will help clarify the patient's concerns. The patient may feel the need to tell you about a problem about his feet while you are listening to his lungs. Take note, and explore the patient's concern without getting sidetracked. The patient will be more cooperative if he feels you are paying attention to this stated concern.

Open, honest, and respectful dialogue with patients and families is a standard of practice for the RN, who is to provide for the safety and security of the patient while respecting rights to privacy and to the integrity of the person. Gaining cooperation from the patient when conducting a nursing action requires the RN to offer a clear explanation, with sound rationale, in advance of the action (FYI 11-8).

Termination Phase

The nurse-patient relationship eventually reaches the final phase, the **termination phase**, the point where the nurse-patient relationship is completed. Completion may be a result of patient discharge or transfer, or of nurse time off or change in employment. Anticipate when this will occur and plan to conclude the relationship that has developed. The termination phase of the nurse-patient relationship needs sufficient planning, time to review goals, and allowance for the patient to recognize that he or she will be able to continue either alone or with the help of another nurse or health care professional.

> ## FYI 11-8 Positive Interviewing Techniques
>
> - The RN who practices sound listening techniques demonstrates a caring attitude.
> - The interview should expand the RN's knowledge of the patient's story.
> - Strong communication is at the level of the patient's understanding, promoting accuracy in the patient's story.
> - Open-ended questions allow patients the opportunity to voice their primary concerns.
> - Focused questioning helps to establish patients' perception of how their health concerns are affecting their life.

With any ending to a relationship, an individual may experience a sense of loss. One characteristic of loss is a feeling of apprehension over the possibility of losing the perceived safety net that has been provided. The patient will need to be supported through the communication efforts of the RN (FYI 11-9). Allow the patient to express fears, and gently point out the progress that has been made. Offering as much information as possible will smooth the course of the termination phase for both the patient and the nurse. If care is to be ongoing, try to prepare the patient and family to establish a relationship with the new caregivers. Make introductions if you are able. See Figure 11-1 for a comparison of timing and phases of communication.

Collaborative Communication

The most difficult form of communication may be when co-workers need to pass information on to one another. To delegate and collaborate with several health care workers, the RN must exercise strong communication skills. As an LPN you have recognized the need for another dimension in communicating with other health care providers. You have been told what to include in your shift reports and charts and what information is

FYI 11-9   Questioning Techniques for the Termination Phase

- Do you remember how far you could walk before you got short of breath? How far can you walk now? What do you think has changed between now and then? *This allows patients to see where they are in relationship to where they were. It also directs the patient to identify those things that might be helping them, such as the medications and the medication schedule. Perhaps a question such as, "What do you think will happen if you forget to take your medication as the doctor has prescribed?" might help the patient identify unacceptable outcomes that could help him or her understand the need for compliance.*

- When I first met you, you were asking for pain medication just about every 2 hours. Tell me how you see your pain control now. *Remember that the patient's story is the most important indicator of how he or she is doing. Pain is subjective, and the nurse cannot assess the level of pain. By listening to the patient's description of his or her pain, the RN can also ask, "What helps you best cope with the pain?" or "What works best to control the pain?"*

- I see that you are beginning to care for your ostomy, emptying and cleaning it. How do you see yourself differently now that you are able to care for yourself? *The patient should express feelings when faced with a significant lifestyle change or image change. The RN who compassionately questions the patient with regard to feelings will gain a better understanding of the patient's progress.*

- Most individuals who have just started giving themselves insulin and checking their sugar levels have a lot of questions. Now that you are giving yourself insulin and are able to do your blood sugar checks, you may still have some questions. What questions do you have? *Acknowledging that it is okay to have questions, even when the patient is expected to be independent in his or her own care, gives the patient permission to not know everything about the process.*

- Right now it must seem a bit puzzling to you, but with time you will know your body's needs, and you will be adjusting your insulin, within the guidelines that the doctor will give you, with confidence. How might you get answers to questions you may have once you leave the hospital? *A statement and question like this one can give reassurance that the patient is progressing as expected and still able to explore available support systems.*

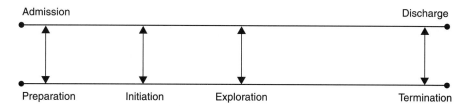

Figure 11-1 Timeline for phases of communication.

important to pass on to the RN, and you can anticipate information the physician wants to know. Although there are LPNs who have leadership roles, most will have been the delegated recipients of information from RNs in charge. Your new role as RN will require many new communication skills.

Delegation

An RN as a care manager needs to delegate many aspects of patient care to many individuals. **Delegation** is the entrusting of a responsibility or task to another who is qualified and who has demonstrated competent ability to carry out the task. A task that can be delegated is one within the scope of practice of the person to whom it has been delegated.

Successful delegation requires sensitive but assertive communication on the part of the RN, which assumes a fair-handed and considerate approach as well as knowing the capabilities and scopes of practice of other staff members. No single simple way exists to ask for cooperation from everyone because each of us is unique and responds to direction in a singular way. The RN who learns to be fair but firm, however, will have greater success in gaining cooperation from more individuals. Consider which of the following requests would be more likely to be followed:

- Request 1: "You need to take that blood pressure and get the reading to me now."

- Request 2: "The blood pressure must be taken right away because I am trying to get through to the physician to get the medication order. I expect that he will get back to me quickly, and the current blood pressure will help him decide what's needed."

Both speakers need the requests completed quickly. Request 1 is more likely to foster resentment since it may be considered aggressive. Request 2 is more respectful yet assertive, and it offers a reason for its urgency.

At times a request may need to be especially firm and exacting, such as when a nurse has not been following directions. This might have been going on for a while. For whatever reason, the LPN, nurse aide, or another RN does not want to follow an important direction or request. In such an instance, the RN in charge eventually needs to find the reason for the resistance, but at the time the request is needed, especially after an explanation has been given, it may be necessary to make the request strongly and to the point. For example, the RN may make the request like this: "I expect that the blood pressure will be done and the results will be given to me before the physician calls back."

Once the urgency of the medical situation has passed and as soon as possible after the incident, the RN needs to ascertain the reason for the resistance. This will take tact as well as assertive communication, which includes being respectful and allowing an explanation to be given. One approach is initially to ask for the seemingly insubordinate individual's own view of the situation: "What was your perception of my request when I first asked you to get a blood pressure on Mr. Smith?" Once this co-worker begins the explanation, the RN should use the same listening skills as would be afforded to a patient's concerns. The nurse should also leave his or her emotions behind, no matter how powerful.

Once you have heard the co-worker out and agree that you have listened, then you can point out how the behavior is getting in the way of giving safe and effective care. If the individual becomes aggressive, then you must recognize the need to stop the conversation and enlist the help of the unit manager or house supervisor, who should be trained to act as a neutral party, in order to arbitrate the situation.

Written Communication

In the course of a day, the nurse needs to communicate in writing on numerous occasions. As an LPN you have learned the importance of patient records as legal documents. As an RN you will be asked to transmit instructions, request equipment, record and explain incidences, and pass on information in writing. In addition to nursing histories and nursing notes, the RN often uses memoranda, e-mail, letters, interdepartmental and interinstitutional forms, and personal diaries or anecdotes to record important information. Each of these forms of written communication must be succinct and accurate.

DOCUMENTATION AS COMMUNICATION The written word becomes a powerful tool that not only contributes to quality patient care but also protects patients, nurses, and the health care agency. The patient's record is documentation establishing that standards of practice, policies, and procedures were followed, and in a legal investigation it can validate that standards of care were met. As a legal document, the patient's chart must be an accurate accounting of the patient's response to the illness and treatment. The nurse must treat the chart as though it will be read in court or at a deposition. Such proceedings often take place more than a few years from the event. The importance of consistently using standard language and approved abbreviations in documentation ensures that if the nurse does need to read the charting and stand behind it at a later date, then he or she will have an easier time in legal matters.

A nurse's notes must be a complete, clear, and relevant record of the patient's course of care. The nurse must chart with consideration of patient outcomes. From the initial assessment to how the patient responds to treatment, continuous evaluation of the patient's condition and the educational needs all form the sequence of the stay within the health care setting. The nursing process formulates the foundation for nursing documentation.

One pitfall to charting is using a medical diagnosis rather than acceptable nursing language to describe a patient condition. Using broad terms instead of specific signs and symptoms opens the nurse to error. For example, an infant with a feeding disorder is given the common medical diagnosis of "dehydration." Describing the infant as dehydrated implies that the nurse has the power to prescribe a medical treatment plan. Nursing documentation should reflect the signs and symptoms assessed that lead the nurse to the conclusion that the infant is dehydrated. The nursing diagnosis of "fluid volume deficit" is within the nursing realm.

When charting, record the patient's exact words verbatim as much as possible, rather than paraphrasing. For example, not many patients would describe their difficulty breathing as "dyspnea," but they may say, "I feel as though I can't catch my breath." Use quotation marks and write exactly what the patient (or family) said that you consider to be relevant.

A common saying is that if you do not chart the nursing or collaborative intervention or the patient response to a treatment, then it did not happen. This implies that all charting must reflect the total nursing process—assessment, diagnosis, outcome identification, planning, implementation, and evaluation—as well as revisions in the plan of care. Common omissions in charting include neglecting to record the patient's response to the interventions, such as whether the patient had pain relief after being given pain medication, or whether the patient had a rhythm change after receiving a cardiac medication. Another common problem with charting is vague or ambiguous terms, such as "worse" and "better." Supplement such patient terms with measures or other quantifications. For example, use a numeric scale to help the patient describe the intensity of pain. Use proper grammar and spelling, not to mention good handwriting. Credibility is maintained when the written word is clear and precise.

In Exercise 11-2, conduct a chart audit, looking at the charting of the nurses in different units. For each nursing entry for a 24-hour period, answer the questions provided. During clinical conference, share the responses with the students in your clinical.

E-mail and memoranda communicate information regarding policy and procedural updates, in-service education, announcements, and patient care. The RN is often asked to respond to such e-mail and memoranda, often to give input or opinion or just to acknowledge having read and understood the message. When a need arises to request services or report patient care concerns to another department, e-mail and memorandum responses will become a challenge for the RN, because the responses will become a record that may be used for or against the writer and are subject to confidentiality issues and federal regulation concerning electronic patient information.

In Exercise 11-3, read the scenario and answer the questions related to memoranda communication.

Official written communications, like oral communication, must be clear and accurate. To ensure clarity and accuracy, include the following elements in your written communication:

- Purpose or need
- Problem or question at issue
- Information, data facts, observations or experiences
- Conclusions or solutions
- Consequences or implications
- Perspective or frame of reference from which the reporting is being made

Exercise 11-2

1. Is the nursing entry dated? _____ Timed? _____ Signed? _____

2. Is the nursing entry legible? _____

3. Are the parts of the nursing process present?

  a. Assessment _____

  b. Diagnosis _____

  c. Outcome Identification _____

  d. Planning _____

  e. Implementation _____

  f. Evaluation _____

4. Was a pain medication given? _____

  a. Did the nurse document the patient's pain intensity? _____ Location? _____

  b. Did the nurse document the patient's response to pain? _____

5. Was a medication given that needed prior special assessment? _____

  a. Did the nurse document the assessment data? _____

  b. Was there a lab value and was it documented? _____

  c. Was the patient's response to the medication documented? _____

6. Was there evidence of patient teaching? _____

  a. Did the nurse document the need for education? _____

  b. What method of education was used?
  Lecture _____ Video _____ Pamphlet _____ Other _____

  c. Did the nurse indicate if there were any special patient considerations? _____

Continued

d. Did the nurse document patient understanding? _____

7. How many spelling and grammatical errors are there? _____

Exercise 11-3

Consider a time when a request for more staff members is made to meet the needs on a specific shift. The data clearly show that acuity levels justify the request, yet the staffing department is unable to find additional staff. After conferring with the supervisor, who is also unable to provide assistance, you become concerned that not all of the care required for the patients will be completed safely and in a timely fashion.

As the RN charge nurse, you will write a memorandum to your unit manager, as well as to the department head, documenting the incidents of the shift. You need to be accurate as well as clear, without being incriminating, in your correspondence.

What information is important to include in the memorandum?

Use this information to create an outline.

How would you avoid demonstrating anger, frustration, or biases, at the same time providing an explanation for specific patient care not being completed?

Each written communication, including occurrence and incident reports, must include an attempt to explain through illustration and examples the importance of the incident to patient safety. In addition, you should make an attempt to maintain neutrality in the reporting, avoiding giving opinion or expressing feelings. Unsafe practice must be reported to division supervisors, facility management, and ultimately the board of nursing. Documentation and correspondence to officials regarding incidences of unsafe practice must be accurate, truthful, and without opinion.

Summary

A different level of exchanging and recording essential information is fundamental to your role change from LPN to RN. Communication must be even more clear, accurate, and fair. The RN is responsible for maintaining ethical and legal integrity with all forms of communication. Personal integrity as well as accountability for the advancement of nursing as a profession requires the RN to excel in all forms of communication. Sound communication skills are a professional standard of practice for the RN. Among the consequences of poor communication are less effective care, low patient satisfaction levels, and unmet or deleterious patient outcomes. A team approach to health care requires the RN to be aware of how he or she communicates with the other team members.

Critical Thinking Questions

The answers to each of the following questions should use the elements of critical thinking: purpose, questions at issue, available information, basic concepts, assumptions, inferences and interpretations, implications and consequences, and point of view.

1. Take a recent clinical situation in which you had a conversation with a patient where there was a need for the patient to understand your point of view in relationship to the plan of care. Write out the conversation, including at least

10 exchanges between you and the patient. From the perspective of sound communication principles, critique your interaction line by line. For each of your statements, give one other way you might have said the same thing and cite a communication principle to back your decision.

2. At report for the beginning of your shift, you find yourself short one staff RN and one nursing aide, according to census data and acuity markers. The staffing office refuses to even look at your request. Though you and your staff make it through the shift and your patients remain safe, you find yourself playing catch-up with charting, and not all the assigned care is complete. A physician is upset that at 7:00 AM his patient's morning weight is not available. Write a memorandum to your unit manager regarding the situation.

3. A new antibiotic medication is being used as part of a clinical trial and is under a strict protocol for administration. The dose for Medication X is to be 1000 units/kg of body weight. The doctor has ordered your patient to receive 100,000 units IVPB over 1 hour. Your patient weighs 125 pounds.

   a. What should be the dose according to the protocol?

   b. Write out what you would say to the physician to get the ordered dosage corrected.

References

Benner P: Nursing leadership for the new millennium: claming the wisdom & worth of clinical practice, *Nurs Health Care Perspect* 20(6):312, 1999.

Benner P, Tanner CA, Chesla CA: *Expertise in nursing practice: caring, clinical judgment, and ethics,* New York, 1996, Springer.

Benner P, Tanner CA, Chesla CA: Becoming an expert nurse, *Am J Nurs* 97(6):16BBB, 1997.

Corbin B: *Identification of family members' self-care knowledge: qualitative study,* MSN thesis, Grand Valley State University, Allendale, Mich, 1990.

Folsom D: Nursing the patient within, *Am J Nurs* 99(7):80, 1999.

Oermann MH: *Professional nursing practice,* Stanford, Conn, 1997, Appleton & Lange.

Taylor C, Lillis C, LeMone P: *Fundamentals of nursing: the art and science of nursing care,* ed 4, Philadelphia, 2001, Lippincott.

Chapter 12

The RN as a Teacher

Key Terms

advocacy
credibility
learning

Overview

An important role of the registered nurse and one defined within state nurse practice acts is the role of teacher. Additionally, a standard of practice expectation is that patient teaching is ultimately the RN's responsibility. The Joint Commission on Accreditation of Healthcare Organizations (JCAHO, 2001) defines the patient education standards to which health care agencies are held accountable. Evidence of performance must demonstrate compliance with these standards for JCAHO accreditation. The implication is that patients have a right to information about their treatment and that a coordinated interdisciplinary effort with patient education needs to exist.

The RN is constantly engaging in both formal and informal patient teaching about some part of care. Education empowers the patient to become active in his or her own health care. The RN needs to understand basic principles of teaching and learning in order to provide the best environment for the patient to learn.

This chapter lays a foundation of sound teaching standards for the student in transition from LPN to RN to develop a teaching plan of care that will empower the patient to be an informed health care consumer and steward of his or her own health. It introduces the student to the principles of learning and to the traits of the adult learner. The chapter presents tools for assessing a patient's readiness to learn and for evaluating the effectiveness of patient education.

The Patient as a Learner

The health care consumer is becoming more informed about health and health care. The consumer is expecting to be educated as to the particular plan of care and to take part in creating that plan. Recent laws and regulations protect consumers by requiring that they receive certain information so that they will be able to make informed choices about their care. JCAHO standards state, "The patient receives education and training specific to the patient's assessed needs, abilities, learning preferences, and readiness to learn as appropriate to the care and services provided by the hospital" (JCAHO, 2001). The JCAHO requires patient education to be interdisciplinary. Furthermore, health care facilities must audit patient education to ensure consistency of teaching and that the health care team members are evaluating the effectiveness of the patient education they give. Just because a consumer received information does not necessarily mean that he or she can demonstrate understanding. The nurse must assess the patient's level of understanding and be prepared to deliver information in a clear and proficient manner.

Principles of Learning

Learning is said to have occurred when a subsequent change in behavior occurs. An informed patient is better able to manage health care, is more compliant with the plan of care, and as a result experiences more positive outcomes. The role of the teacher is important, and mastery of the role is essential to professional practice. As a teacher, you will advocate for the patient by giving the information needed to make decisions. **Advocacy** means to promote an idea, belief, or person or to put someone in the best possible position to assist himself or herself. As a patient advocate, you will use your teaching skills as a means to empower patients toward healthier lifestyles.

Basic Assumptions of Learning

You have chosen to return to school to learn what is needed to become an RN. You have chosen the opportunity to learn by enrolling in and attending classes. Interestingly, although students recognize the need for additional knowledge and experience, they often question the necessity of some of the readings and other material presented in class or clinical. You may question the need to study particular assigned material and choose to concentrate on material that seems more important for a test. Given this, two basic assumptions for learning are important for the individual to understand:

1. Individuals choose to learn or not to learn.
2. What the individual perceives as important is more readily learned.

In the health care setting, patients are seldom given a choice about whether they need to learn. RNs, LPNs, physicians, and other health care workers generally dictate what each patient needs to know. They will either direct the teaching or present the teaching material without consulting the patient. Often this includes little or no assessment of the patient's learning needs. For example, patients with newly diagnosed insulin-dependent diabetes mellitus will be given lessons on how to monitor their glucose levels and to give themselves insulin. Even so, many patients return to the acute care setting with complications related to "noncompliance" with their new regimens. When questioned, the patients often do not remember anyone telling them how to deal with their new diagnosis in great detail.

Much of what is presented as patient education ignores basic principles of learning. Patients may not be in a condition to learn. Furthermore, unless the patient clearly states it, he or she may not understand the relevance of the information to the condition. In general, where patient education is concerned, more is better than less, and multiple methods of presenting information will increase the likelihood that your patient will retain it.

Motivation to Learn

Individuals inherently hold to their own values and beliefs as truths until they have significant motivation to change. The motivation to learn often results from a life-changing event, such as childbirth or illness. A patient may perceive learning as an opportunity to improve the condition or make a difference in another significant way. The RN who recognizes the significance of the event can seize the opportunity to explore the patient's motivation to learn.

Barriers to Learning

Myths and misconceptions about health, illness, and health care are often perpetuated by the experiences of the individual. The patient who has had knowledge of someone dying from a particular disorder is more likely to see the disorder in a dismal light and be willing to accept statistics that support a bleak picture. The nurse may have difficulty convincing the patient that his or her particular prognosis is actually more optimistic. The opposite may also be true. A patient with the same disorder but who has known someone who got better and lived long and healthy may not be as willing to accept statistics showing that the disorder may have a bleak outcome. For example, despite the amount of hard evidence showing a positive relationship between cigarette smoking and a multitude of health problems, many people are not willing to believe it. This way of thinking is known as *denial*.

Patient values influence the willingness to accept the need to change and therefore the need to learn. Patients whose values are contrary to the evidence will need to have time to understand the relevance of the information that you are giving them. The smoker will need time to understand that a relationship exists between his or her symptoms and smoking. Therefore the RN must use rational thought and convey that logic in the presentation of the facts. The patient must decide that the change is necessary. The RN can only act as a conduit of knowledge and for rational thought, leaving prejudices, feelings, and frustrations behind. You may need to set up a referral for further assistance. In any case, you must understand the patient's decision and show acceptance of it.

Facilitation of Learning

Other general principles of learning should be considered when engaging patients in the learning process. FYI 12-1 outlines some of the principles that facilitate learning. The RN must understand that learning takes place in segments and that a patient can absorb only so much, or reach a

---

FYI 12-1 Facilitators to Learning

A learner:

- Is motivated to make a change in life.
- Believes that the information to be learned will be beneficial.
- Believes that it is possible to learn what is needed.
- Has clear and reasonable outcome objectives.
- Has a low to moderate level of stress.
- Has had other immediate needs met.
- Believes that the changes related to learning will have a positive influence on his or her life.

plateau, before the learning process becomes ineffective. These plateaus often do not correspond with the goals and outcomes set by the nurse. When a patient has reached a plateau, the behavior may be labeled as lazy, noncompliant, or difficult to manage. The RN must remember that true learning is a life-changing event, and change is stressful. A patient being asked, or forced by necessity, to go through a lot of change at one time can put up resistance. Positive reinforcement for the change that has taken place, rather than negative feedback as to what the patient still needs to learn, will maintain a trusting relationship, which will foster continued learning.

Understanding how the learning process occurs will help the RN plan teaching sessions. If the patient is involved in the process of planning and active in learning, a better patient outcome is inevitable.

Adult Learners

Adult patients are adult learners. Adults bring to the health care setting a lifetime of experiences that will influence how they perceive formal and informal learning. Assessment of a patient's life experiences will help you plan learning activities. The closer the learning can be applied to the patient's past experiences, the easier it is for the patient to accept the need to learn and thus to change behavior.

Eduard Lindeman (1926), one of the founding fathers of the theory of adult learning, made five important assumptions about adult learners that may serve to guide the nurse's efforts at patient education:

1. Adults will learn as they develop needs that they believe learning will fulfill.
2. Adults use their lives as the point of reference for all learning.
3. Adults learn best from and in relation to their experiences.
4. Adults prefer to be self-directed in learning, or at the very least have a say in it.
5. Differences between individuals broaden with age and experience.

Relating to the Learner's Level of Understanding

Adults need new information to be related to something they already know. This creates a link so that the information can be readily recalled. For example, compliance with fluid restriction may be easier if you as a nurse create an analogy or familiar frame of reference. Most adults will be able to relate to the heart and blood vessels in household plumbing terms. Compare the heart to a sump pump that must run in order for a basement not to fill up with water. When this concept is applied to the need for the heart to pump effectively so the lungs will not fill up with water, the patient may better understand congestive heart failure. Additionally, the individual will understand the need not to add to the water in the basement and that this concept applies to not adding to the water in the lungs.

In many cases, institutions provide written instructions to patients in the hope that they will use them as references. Studies have shown that a lower-than-expected level of literacy may exist in patient populations seeking health care within the United States, as reported in a search by Fisher (1999). A report from the Ad Hoc Committee on Health Literacy for the Council on Scientific Affairs, American Medical Association (1999), concluded that "patients with the greatest health care needs may have the least ability to read and comprehend information needed to function successfully as patients" (p. 552). The implication for nursing of this and other studies is that the RN should recognize that patients may not have the comprehension of material needed to manage their own care. Simply asking patients whether they understand may not be enough to ensure that understanding is adequate.

A need exists to design further research that will include literacy and comprehension assessment tools. Providing literature without knowing the level of the patient's ability to understand may put the patient at risk for further health complications. A review of current patient education literature, consent forms, and discharge instruction sheets may be necessary to assess the reading level. Recommendations may need to be made to adjust material to ensure that as many patients as possible are served. FYI 12-2 provides general learning principles for adult patients.

In Exercise 12-1, read the scenario and answer the questions concerning an adult learner's level of understanding.

Assessment of Readiness to Learn

Two assumptions we often make when educating is that the patient has benefited from the experience and learning has taken place. The reality is often the opposite because the patient will be under stress from the medical problem as well as the environment, and the addition of a learning experience would add to the stress. The patient may be motivated to learn

FYI 12-2   General Principles of Learning

- Individuals will learn in response to perceived needs. A sound teaching plan is designed from the assessed learning needs of the patient.

- Active learning (being able to direct and assist in assessing and pianning learning) facilitates the learning process. An RN who recognizes the need for the patient to be an active learner will gain trust and empower the patient to take charge of health care concerns.

- If the material to be learned has meaning to the individual, learning is easier. Concepts or ideas form the foundation for learning facts, procedures, and rules.

- Learning that has direct application or use for the individual will be retained longer. Assessment of the patient's understanding of the health concerns in relation to his or her experiences will help you design a teaching plan that is empathetic to the patient's individual needs.

- A patient who can see progress is motivated to learn more.

- Mild anxiety enhances learning, yet moderate to severe anxiety detracts from the learning process.

- Patients come to the health care setting with a lifetime of learning experiences. If learning can be associated with relevant real-life experiences, then the patient has a greater chance for retention of the material.

Exercise 12-1

RN: It must be difficult for you to quit smoking.

Patient: I have been smoking all my life, and I don't plan on stopping just because my doctor has told me to.

RN: What has the doctor told you about smoking and the problems you are having?

Patient: He said that my breathing will get better if I stop smoking. I find that hard to believe because when I have a cigarette, I tend to feel more relaxed, and my breathing becomes easier. I have the hardest time in the morning when I haven't had a cigarette all night.

RN: Are there other times when you have difficulty breathing?

Patient: Yes, but only when I exert myself more than normal, like walking up a flight of stairs. I just use elevators when I can.

RN: So, you find the times you have the most difficulty are when you awaken and when you exert yourself. When was the last time you can remember not having difficulty with your breathing in the morning?

Patient: Oh, I suppose it was when I was younger, maybe in my twenties. I was in good shape then. I have gotten older, I guess less fit.

RN: So, you were more fit when you were in your twenties, and now that you are in your fifties, you feel less fit?

Patient: Yes, I guess so. I get around all right. This blasted pneumonia was unexpected.

RN: Do you think you are having more or less difficulty than other men your age have with their breathing?

Patient: Oh, I know a few people who are like me, and I know some who are in better shape. I think I am like my father; he had lung problems and died of them.

1. What type of prejudicial thinking does this patient have that the RN will need to overcome?

2. What further questions could be asked of the patient to assist him toward a better understanding of his problem?

Continued

3. What would the nursing diagnosis "knowledge deficit" be related to in this scenario?

4. What would the nursing diagnosis "denial" be related to in this scenario?

5. What would be another nursing diagnosis?

yet not ready to learn. Readiness for learning must be assessed before beginning the teaching process (FYI 12-3)

Understanding Stressors

The number of stresses on the patient will influence the patient's ability to understand and remember new information. Take, for example, a patient entering a same-day surgery center. The time frame before the surgery, or for any procedure, is typically short; yet the standard of care requires the RN to teach the patients about the care. The patient should

---

FYI 12-3 **Factors Conducive to Successful Learning**

- Learning takes place when behavior has changed. Change is stressful, and if the patient is experiencing additional stress, learning will be compromised.
- An RN must assess a patient's readiness to learn.
- The patient must be in the best possible condition before a teaching session.
- The family can assist the patient in the learning process.
- The patient's environment must be prepared before a teaching session.
- The patient who becomes an expert in his or her own care is empowered to maintain physical and psychological well-being.

---

understand several elements of the impending surgery. The RN will also need to teach the patient about his or her active participation in the recovery process (for example, cough and deep breathing exercises or pain control methods). In many instances, after the procedure the patient forgets what was said because true learning did not occur.

How can such a situation be avoided? In an outpatient surgical setting, teaching is typically done at the physician's office sometime before the procedure. Providing written material in advance of the day of surgery will give the patient time to read and understand the information.

Need to Include Family in the Learning Process

Family members and close friends can be assets to the RN during a patient teaching session. They will be able to reinforce the patient's education. Family members may advocate for loved ones, seek clarification, and act as coaches to encourage compliance with health care teaching. Often their need for information will be met as a result of their inclusion in the education sessions. Be certain, however, to assess the accuracy of the family's understanding of what you present.

Assess the Patient's Current Level of Knowledge

Some patients are experts in regard to their ailment. A lot of information is available about illnesses and treatments, and with the advent of the Internet, this information is even more readily available. This means that the patient entering the health care system may be well informed and have expectations for care. Such a patient has taken control of his or her life by learning as much as possible and incorporating it into elements of daily care. Hutchings (1999) described, through a case study, the importance of developing a health-promoting plan of care for a chronic illness by recognizing patients as experts. According to Hutchings, getting all patients to this expert position is important as a means of empowering them to better master their environment by maintaining both physical and psychological well-being.

To avoid or correct errors, determine the accuracy of information the patient provides about the condition. Not only are many reliable resources of medical information available but many unreliable, untested sources, as well. Ask the patient where the information came from.

Evaluation of Effectiveness of Learning

The RN must verify that learning, not just teaching, has taken place (FYI 12-4; Exercise 12-2). For learning to have occurred, the patient must incorporate the learned behavior into his or her life. Assessment of the patient's learning is often completed at the time the teaching is done, yet in reality an assessment done a day or two later may be a better indicator of the retention and incorporation of new information or behavior changes.

FYI 12-4 Evaluation of Learning

- The RN must be able to demonstrate that learning has taken place.

- The RN must take into consideration the literacy levels of the patient when evaluating learning and the patient's level of knowledge.

- More research needs to take place regarding effectiveness of patient teaching.

Legal Implications

While the standard of care is for the RN to be aware of the learning needs of the patient and provide a plan of care that will meet those needs, the RN often has difficulty demonstrating that learning has taken place. The standard of care dictates that patient teaching include information regarding both the disorder and the treatment plan. The legal and ethical consequences of not providing and/or documenting that learning has occurred may place the RN in a position of being accused of inability to provide safe patient care.

Demonstration of Learning

Demonstration of learning can take place when a patient is observed completing a task without complications or consequences. The skill of a patient or family member who must do dressing changes at home can be observed and evaluated for effectiveness. The patient's understanding of the concept of sterility or of hypoglycemia, for example, is more difficult for the

Exercise 12-2

Two patients have been taught about their dietary restrictions with regard to their newly diagnosed diabetes mellitus. Each is being assessed for understanding of the limitations to diet.

Patient One: When I take my DiaBeta in the morning, I am free to eat what I want during the day. I will be glad not to have to be on the diet I was on before. It's okay for me to keep some hard candies in case the DiaBeta causes my blood sugar to go too low. In fact, I think I should eat one every now and then just to keep from getting too low.

Patient Two: I know that the DiaBeta will help me keep my blood sugar down if I stay with my diet. I am concerned about the times that I might get low blood sugar levels. Should I carry some sort of candy with me for those times, or should I use something else instead? It is hard for me to know just what to do.

Which patient would need further teaching?

RN to assess. The RN may need to request an order for home health visits to follow up on patient teaching. A home health nurse can reassess the patient's knowledge and determine the need for further teaching.

A return demonstration of a procedure one time does not mean the patient has achieved understanding. RNs and LPNs have a way of coaching patients through a procedure and then documenting that the patients "demonstrated understanding." Avoid words that cannot be measured, such as "understanding." When you are documenting, all that you can record is that the patient was able to demonstrate the procedure and followed the basic principles at the time of observation. To state that the patient demonstrated understanding as a result of one observation would be incorrect because many factors are present at the time of the observation that may influence the patient's ability to understand.

Following Up After Discharge

Another method to evaluate effectiveness of patient learning may be a call system, where the patient receives a telephone call from the RN 2 or 3 days after discharge. The RN will assess the patient's condition and need for further instruction. Careful assessment questions can identify problems and uncover teaching needs that have not been met. The RN will then revise the teaching plan to include areas of patient need and provide for follow-up if an assessed need exists.

Characteristics of a Teacher

You have had teachers who made an impression on you, as either motivating and skilled or boring and dictatorial. You have perhaps attended conferences where one of the speakers was so inspiring that you may have made a change. Among several important characteristics of successful teachers are credibility, confidence, and the ability to communicate effectively.

Nurse Credibility

Credibility implies that the nurse has credentials or licensure and is honest enough to fulfill duties to the fullest and best of his or her ability. The RN has basic and advanced knowledge of how to decrease the risk factors for many diseases as well as how to promote a wellness state. A fundamental concept of the role of teacher is the maintenance of current knowledge of all aspects of patient care within the specialty. Knowledge must be practiced as well and taught by example. Many nurses do not practice wellness habits themselves and thus have difficulty promoting wellness habits in their patients. The nurse who is a smoker yet teaches patients about smoking cessation, for example, will not be as credible as one who has quit smoking or never smoked.

Need for Confidence

The RN must communicate effectively with confidence and be well prepared with the material to be presented. The RN must have knowledge and skill and present it as a credible source. A teacher needs to speak clearly and precisely for the patient to gain from the learning experience. Practice is important for patient teaching to be effective. Because teacher is a role that the RN assumes on a daily basis, he or she should make the effort to hone this skill. Knowing the basics of adult learning and ensuring the patient's readiness to learn will assist in preparation for teaching, but to deliver a message effectively, you should practice interpersonal communication skills.

To improve at teaching, you should critique yourself. A self-evaluation journal is one way to look at what worked and what you could have done differently. A self-evaluation should take place as soon as you exit the teaching experience or as soon as possible before the end of the day.

Clear and Effective Communication

Clear, precise communication skills are fundamental to teaching. Terminology that is well defined and understood by the patient is a major consideration. For example, an RN may explain about the patient's heart failure, talking about how sodium intake causes osmosis to occur in the kidneys, resulting in pulmonary edema. In this scenario at least four or five terms would be difficult for the patient to comprehend. When asked to comply with the dietary restrictions, the patient may then be too confused to understand what is needed. Adjust your explanations such that your patient education is delivered clearly, accurately, and in understandable terms.

Tools of the Teacher

To ensure that the patient and family are ready to learn, the RN must prepare the learning environment. As much privacy as possible can help ensure that the patient and family are comfortable discussing the treatment plan.

Minimize distractions and noise by asking that the television be turned off. Provide privacy by selecting a private location or excusing roommates or certain family members. Ensure that the patient has received medications that help him or her feel well, and delay (if advisable) medication that may cause distracting side effects, such as nausea or drowsiness. The RN should be positioned to deliver teaching comfortably, while looking relaxed and interested in the process rather than stressed or hurried. Teaching can often take place while the RN is seated next to the patient.

To assist in the learning process, the RN should have appropriate teaching aids ready. A model of the heart, kidney, or central line, for example, will help the patient picture the procedure or condition. The patient can also view a video, and the RN will then be available to answer questions and clarify the content.

Pamphlets can be good resources for the patient, again leaving the RN to clarify or expand on the content. An obvious determination to make before offering reading material is that the patient be able to read it, so the RN must assess the patient's reading level. Most health-related reading material is at the 6th- through 8th-grade level, but not all patients will read even that well. Including family members by offering them the pamphlets may be helpful because they may be able to assist the patient in reading comprehension. Reading material must also be in the appropriate language for the patient; a patient who reads only Spanish will not be able to learn much from a pamphlet in English. Your patient may require pamphlets written in Braille or audiotapes.

You should also consider the learning style of the individual patient. For example, some people learn best by practice or hands-on experiences. Others learn by reading or by listening to a lecture. Providing a variety of ways to deliver the information—by video, demonstrations, pamphlets, and more—will assist each learner in understanding and retaining the information.

Summary

The RN is constantly engaging in formal and informal patient teaching. The RN must practice basic principles of teaching and understand the fundamentals of adult learning. A standard of care is for the RN to engage in patient teaching. Effective teaching can empower the patient to better manage his or her own health care, become more compliant with the plan of care, and have more positive outcomes.

Critical Thinking Questions

1. Identify a teaching need in a patient for whom you are to care. Design a simple teaching plan that includes the following:

   - How you will assess the patient for a teaching need
   - The identified teaching need
   - Information you will need to gather to teach the topic, including references from at least two sources
   - Where the teaching will take place
   - Props, audiovisuals, or reading material you will need
   - How you will prepare the environment to optimize learning
   - How much time you will need to teach
   - Data that support the patient's readiness to learn
   - Measures you will take to evaluate whether learning has taken place
   - Evaluation of the teaching and a self-evaluation of your ability as a teacher

2. A patient is to receive an experimental treatment. The doctor has been in to explain the procedure, and the patient has signed the consent form. In doing an assessment before the procedure, the patient states, "I really didn't understand what the doctor told me, except he said I should get better. I hope I do get better."

   a. What is your responsibility as an RN at this point?

b. What questions would you ask the patient at this time?

c. What questions would you ask your supervisor or manager if the patient had significant discomfort about the impending procedure?

3. You are to give an in-service on one of the cardiogenic medications and explain to a new group of RNs how to measure the medication by µg/kg/min. For patients who are 160 lb, 110 lb, and 205 lb, and for the following doctor's order, figure the correct mg/min pump setting.

a. Order reads for Medication A to run at 5 µg/kg/min. It is available as 50 mg in 250 ml of D_5W.

b. Order reads for Medication B to run at 10 µg/kg/min. It is available as 1 g in 500 ml of NS.

c. Medication C is available as 500 mg in 250 ml of D_5W. The pump is running at 20 ml/min. What is the dose?

References

Ad Hoc Committee on Health Literacy for the Council on Scientific Affairs, American Medical Association: Health literacy: report of the Council on Scientific Affairs, *JAMA* 281(6):552, 1999.

Fisher E: Low literacy levels in adults: implications for patient education, *J Contin Educ Nurs* 30(2):56, 1999.

Hutchings D: Partnership in education: an example of client and educator collaboration, *J Contin Educ Nurs* 30b(3):128, 1999.

Joint Commision on Accreditation of Healthcare Organizations: *2001 hospital accreditation standards,* Oakbrook Terrace, IL, 2001, Author.

Lindeman EC: *The meaning of adult education,* New York, 1926, New Republic.

Chapter 13

The RN as a Manager of Care

Key Terms

accountability
advocacy
collaboration
conflict
interpersonal conflict
leadership

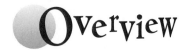verview

Being a manager of care is a major role of the RN, who is expected to become primarily responsible for managing the plan of care for several patients. As an LPN, you already have basic management skills that will assist you in understanding the coordinator of care role. You will be not only a well-organized coordinator but also a collaborator within a team to deliver safe, effective care.

This chapter presents leadership characteristics and styles as well as other components of your new role, such as task delegation, conflict management, accountability, and advocacy for care. It also explores discharge planning.

Leadership Characteristics

Implementation of the plan of care for several patients takes organization and **leadership**, the ability to influence outcomes through positive interactions with team members. A strong leader recognizes the strengths and weaknesses within the team and manages them to effect a positive outcome from a plan of care. Morrison, Jones, and Fuller (1997) contend that an important aspect of leadership is empowerment of all the team members to do the jobs of which they are most capable.

Defining the Leadership Role

Basic to the leadership role is the ability to know the defined roles of each team member, as well as their strengths and weakness. A strong leader delegates assignments, tasks, and duties to the best individuals for the particular jobs. A strong leader empowers the team members through delegation of tasks within their capacity and by the trust placed in them to complete these tasks. Morrison, Jones, and Fuller (1997) conclude that job satisfaction increases when there is empowerment. Laschinger and colleagues (1999) suggest that a leader's empowerment behavior predicts a lower level of job tension and more effective work.

To *manage* is directing or supervising others as a means to control a situation (Marquise and Huston, 2000). Managing patient care means overseeing the plan of care and directing others to implement the plan toward achievement of the desired outcomes. A manager has leadership qualities, acts as an advisor, and influences the beliefs of others. With the RN as a patient care manager, the leadership role is both an expectation as well as an earned role. It is an assumption that a strong leader has expertise in the practice area or clinical specialty. A strong leader knows about the patients and is able to anticipate their needs. Within this role, the RN is confident, in control of the day, and willing to help when needed.

The RN leader is decisive, practices sound judgment, and is able to articulate fluently. Perra (1999) associates a sound leader with self-knowledge, respect, trust, integrity, vision, participation, learning, communication, and catalyzing change. Respect and trust are mutual and inclusive between the leader and team members. Respect comes to the leader with integrity, who reliably does the right thing by all and for the profession. Leadership fosters participation from others in the critical thinking process, as sources of information, expertise, and specific knowledge. The leader with integrity advocates diversity of opinion and beliefs within the team and is thus open to critiques of actions and decisions.

The strong leader is a critical and rational thinker. Such an RN leader is better equipped to influence the other health care team members and gain their cooperation and respect.

Leadership Styles

Leadership styles emerge as ways to relate to others and influence the outcomes of situations. Each style has distinct qualities that define it and make it suitable for meeting a particular situation's team objectives. The three main styles are democratic, autocratic, and laissez-faire leadership. You need to know when to use which leadership type, based on your assessment of the situation:

- The *democratic leader* bases decisions on *consensus,* or mutual agreement, within the group. This leader delegates duties according to the strengths within the team. With each team member solicited for input, however, outcomes are slow in coming.

- Authoritarian and *autocratic leaders* use power to influence others and effect outcomes. If the autocratic leader just assumes power without earning the subordinates' respect, though, that power can foster resentment. Authoritarian power exerted in an acute crisis situation, however, can effectively influence outcomes.

- A *laissez-faire*, or nondirective, *leader* deliberately intervenes as little as possible. When team members are independently motivated yet cohesive, much can be accomplished over a period of time. Chaos can occur, however, if individual needs and agendas interfere with the overall goals of the group.

Additionally, a group may have more than one leader, requiring either a co-leadership approach or a rotating leadership approach. The dynamics of the group as well as the individual leaders generally dictate the success of such a group.

Leadership has been described in relationship to either a transactional or a transformational style, influencing change through empowerment of the nurse and team members (Morrison, Jones, and Fuller, 1997; Trofino, 1995). A transactional leader leads through cost-benefit or some economic reward exchange with a subordinate. The transformational leader uses characteristics such as inspiration, charisma, intellectual stimulation, and idealized influence to effect a change in the subordinate (Morrison, Jones, and Fuller, 1997). The transformational leader influences change through empowering the followers to do the work of change. Within a group process, this leadership style supports the competencies of the individual members, allowing them to take responsibility and authority for their decisions. This leadership style fosters support for creativity, uniqueness in problem solving, and an individual spirit of freedom. Team members feel empowered to do their work and often perform at a higher level than expected. Fundamental trust is established between leader and follower, and the task of the team is fulfilled with a high degree of patient satisfaction.

Choosing a Style

The RN's style of leadership should reflect the personalities of the group members as well as respond to the situation. Individual personalities affect the group interaction. A strong leader understands such dynamics and capitalizes on them. An example might be when the RN is determining patient assignments. Knowing the personalities of the group, the RN makes assignments so that each member will use his or her best attributes and best work together with the others. For example, an RN team leader could assign an LPN who does not need much direction to be supervised by an RN who is known to expect independence from the LPNs. In another example, the RN team leader may make patient assignments based on the critical nature of the situation, delegating critical patient care to the most experienced RN.

Generally, the RN as a manager of care incorporates one or more styles of leadership to meet the needs of the patient. Judicious leadership takes open communication between the group members. Clear goals and objectives must be a part of the plan of care, and each member of the team must understand his or her role in meeting the goals. When a team works together for a common goal, communicating positive patient outcomes and patient satisfaction to the team members can give a sense of pride and accomplishment (Morrison, Jones, and Fuller, 1997).

Collaborator in Providing Care

Collaboration is a partnership arrangement between two or more individuals where there is mutual agreement to work together. Each partner brings to the group unique talents and skills, which will be used to create the best possible outcome or to meet specific goals. The RN, recognizing that the health care team is made up of unique individuals, takes into account the many resources available, such as these specific skills and knowledge, when designing the plan of care. Some concepts related to the collaborator of care role are delegation, accountability, advocacy, and respect for self and for other health care workers.

Delegation of Care

Delegation is the process of assigning tasks or duties to an entrusted individual. Marquis and Huston define delegation as "getting work done through others or as directing the performance of one or more people to accomplish organizational goals" (2000, p. 330). Appropriate delegation requires the RN to base judgments on who is most qualified for the job. An RN inherently does not know, but must learn, the job descriptions or the state board limitations on the LPN or the state regulations of unlicensed personal. The LPN or health care aide is then an assumed representative of the RN, acting under the authority of the RN. The LPN or health care aide is expected to report to the RN the results of the intervention as well as the patient's response.

When delegating tasks, interventions, and duties to other team members, the RN must always maintain patient safety. The RN must therefore understand the scopes of practice of the LPNs, health care aides, respiratory care therapist, and everyone else on the health care team, not just their knowledge and skill levels.

The RN must respect each team member and be respected by them for delegation to be effective. The RN will build trust and be appreciated because of consistent, appropriate delegation, encouragement, and compassionate understanding of each team member. Take, for example, the RN who appears to consistently make patient assignments to minimize his or her own workload. When others are working hard to get through the day, this RN does not offer support or assistance but, rather, is seen to be spending time doing comparatively very little. In contrast, consider the RN who both delegates difficult assignments to appropriate individuals and has an equally difficult assignment or is available to assist the other team members. This RN will be a highly regarded team leader, gain more cooperation from the others, and experience greater patient satisfaction and positive patient outcomes.

Delegating fairly does not mean delegating equally. The leader bases assignments on individual capability, which means the experienced RN's assignment may be challenging and the inexperienced RN's relatively less challenging. Every member of the team should understand the role, capacity, and responsibility of every other member. As the experience level of the team members equalizes, so too will the assignments.

The lead RN may have difficulty communicating apparent assignment disparities to all the team members involved. If the RN shows understanding of this while helping the others recognize the differences between them, this may facilitate cooperation. However, the RN must be alert to a potential for conflict and use the skills presented in the following section to head off or resolve conflict.

Conflict Management

Conflict is an opposition of feelings, beliefs, desires, or goals. Conflict is generally considered to be a negative occurrence or state, yet in reality it is neutral since either positive or negative outcomes can result. Conflict can be intrapersonal, within one individual; interpersonal, between two or more individuals; intragroup, within one group; or intergroup, between two or more groups (Marquis and Huston, 2000; Smith, 1992; Sullivan and Decker, 1988). The individual and group responses to conflict may create problems within the workplace. A conflict has a preceding causative event, which sets up a perceived or felt antagonism. Conflict within the health care workplace becomes a source of discord when a disruption occurs in patient care activities. Examples of possible causative events are staffing mixes, ethical decisions, and punitive measures. Perceived differences in care management, patient load responsibility, and personality differences can also be sources of conflict between the RN coordinator of patient care and others on the care team. Lack of mutual respect between the RN and the others may result from unresolved conflict.

Conflict management is a challenging skill that the RN must master in order to lead a team in the role of manager of care (FYI 13-1). You can learn and practice basic principles of conflict management, such as sacrifice resolution, competition resolution, and win-win resolution.

SACRIFICE RESOLUTION   When two people compromise to resolve conflict, they both give up their positions. Neither gets exactly what he or she wants, but both are able to live with the decision. Conversely, in sacrifice resolution one may strongly want to avoid or end the conflict and will therefore accommodate the other by essentially sacrificing his or her position, thus allowing the other to have his or her way. The one who continually sacrifices in order to accommodate others may build up resentment that could eventually surface inappropriately.

COMPETITION RESOLUTION   Another form of conflict resolution is when one or both of the parties work competitively, instead of cooperatively, toward resolution. The problem with resolving conflicts in this manner is that one side wins and the other loses. The obvious result is resentment or jealousy on the part of the individual who lost. An example of this type of conflict resolution is when a unit manager posts a memo regarding holiday or vacation schedule requests. If clear rules are not in place that direct a fair distribution of days off among the staff members, certain individuals may view this as an opportunity to "win" their preferred days off at the expense of others. A policy of "first come, first served" would be unfair in this situation. In that case, staff members working the shift when the schedule comes out would be in

FYI 13-1   **Steps to Collaborative Conflict Resolution**

1. Open a dialogue that brings forth and is respectful of each individual's point of view.

2. Determine a group or shared goal.

3. Identify the expertise and contribution of each individual as the group agrees upon the shared goal.

4. Review the goal and move to honestly accept or reject it (acceptance requires the consensus of the group).

5. Design a plan to meet the new goal, using the expertise of the group to design interventions to meet the goal.

6. Determine the roles of the members in carrying out the interventions. A role must be within the capacity of the member and mutually accepted as fairly defined.

7. Set an evaluation point and include all individuals in the evaluation process. Maintain respect for everyone's input or contribution, as well as focusing on interventions and actions, rather than personalities, feelings, or prejudices.

a better position to request days off before others who are not there. This practice of competitive conflict resolution pits staff members against one another and creates resentment toward the manager as well as toward the individuals who take advantage of it.

WIN-WIN RESOLUTION   Setting up a win-win situation requires a collaborative method of conflict resolution (Marquis and Houston, 2000). The two opposing parties come together to decide on mutual goals, design interventions to meet these goals, and work together to evaluate the outcomes. Because the parties agree on how to deal with the situation, all parties involved have a sense of ownership and will generally work together to achieve the best outcome for all. Engaging in collaborative steps to resolve conflict may assist the RN in managing conflicts that threaten to derail the team and ultimately impede patient care. If the example in the previous section were handled with win-win resolution, the manager might post the memo with a deadline for sign-up and then hold a staff meeting to discuss it.

INTERPERSONAL CONFLICT **Interpersonal conflict**, or conflict between two or more people, may need a more immediate approach to resolution because it may result in compromised patient care. The first steps are for the RN to recognize that those involved each have points of view worth considering, think through each point of view in a logical manner, and ask the parties to assist in helping to clarify the issues. An assertive, logical, and reasoned approach is necessary for assessing the situation. The RN must not act with emotion but always stay focused on the facts of the issue, or more importantly on the potential consequences for patient safety if resolution were not to occur. The RN must also articulate his or her own point of view as team leader in an equally clear and rational manner.

The RN may need to be autocratic if the situation is critical and the behavior of one of the parties is impeding timely resolution of a patient problem. In a less critical situation, the RN may have more time for a more collaborate approach. A win-win situation can occur if the RN is willing to work toward common goals and objectives, rather than just putting forth his or her own agenda. Exercise 13-1 illustrates an interpersonal conflict situation between an RN and an aide.

Any discussion regarding conflict should be done in an area that gives as much privacy as possible, especially away from patient care areas where patients or families may overhear the discussion. The key focus must be on patient care and patient care safety. Both parties must be willing to talk calmly and rationally. If the other party is angry and out of control, then you must stop the discussion. You can then explain that you will take the discussion up at a later time. If and when you cannot resolve a conflict, you must know when to stop and recruit a manager to assist.

Accountability for Care

The RN as coordinator of care is accountable for patient outcomes as they apply to the plans of care for the patients. When delegating responsibilities to the team members or collaborating with other departments to extend care, the RN must evaluate the effectiveness of the plan of care.

Exercise 13-1

A new RN on a busy medical-surgical unit is attempting to direct a patient care aide who is being argumentative and disruptive with regard to her patient care assignment. The health care aide has refused to assist a patient with ambulating, complaining that RNs have learned to ambulate patients, and he should do it, not her. The RN needs the aide to complete vital signs on a new surgical patient each hour over the next 3 hours as well as ambulate a patient who is 2 days postoperation. The following conversation takes place between the RN and the health care aide in the breakroom:

RN: You have stated that you refuse to ambulate the patient in room 769. Help me understand your reason for refusal.

Health care aide: You're new to this floor; what gives you the authority to tell me what I'm supposed to do? You've been taught how to walk a patient; I think you should walk him.

RN: How is my role different from that of the other RNs?

Health care aide: You need to know your place on this floor. I have more experience than you. I know my job; I do it well. You don't need to tell me what to do.

1. What is the health care aide's main issue?

2. What is the best way for the RN to proceed with resolving this conflict?

3. What is the priority of care that the RN should remember in dealing with this conflict?

Accountability means the RN must ensure that the medical and nursing plan of care is implemented, evaluated, and possibly modified so that the patient outcomes are the best they possibly can be.

The RN is accountable for delegating inappropriately. That is, if the RN knowingly delegates an assignment beyond someone's qualifications or scope of practice, then the RN assumes responsibility for any negative consequences. For example, an RN gives a medication to a health care aide with instructions to make sure that the patient takes it. The health care aide, not instructed in the five rights, fails to identify the patient correctly, which results in giving the medication to the wrong patient, who is harmed. The coordinating RN has clearly failed to follow standards of practice as well as policies and the nurse practice act. The RN should be reprimanded and risks sanctions from the board of nursing.

Many situations regarding delegation and accountability are not completely clear, yet the RN must be aware of conditions, however subtle, that will place patients at risk. For example, the RN delegates a patient's dressing change to an LPN who has learned sterile technique and can do dressing changes. The patient develops a wound infection, however. If the RN had not adequately assessed the wound, only relying on the LPN's assessment, and knew the patient was at risk for developing an infection, then the RN failed to render safe care, neglecting a fundamental duty to the patient.

Job descriptions, policies, procedures, and licensure dictate the roles and responsibilities of each member of the team. The RN is not accountable for the LPN or health care aide who willfully neglects a patient or steps over the bounds of legal limitations. Whoever is acting in a reckless or neglectful manner is responsible. For example, the LPN who makes a medication error is responsible for the error, unless the error was made in collaboration with the RN. In any case, the RN would be accountable for taking steps to minimize the effects of the negligence, document the incident, and appropriately communicate the incident per hospital policy and procedure as well as board of nursing guidelines.

Advocate for Care

Advocacy occurs when one individual promotes someone else or someone's idea. As a patient advocate, the RN promotes the patient's decisions in a nonjudgmental manner. By being involved in the plan of care, the patient is informed and can express feelings and preferences. Additionally, the RN should know what the physician tells the patient with regard to the condition and treatment plan. If possible, the RN makes rounds with the physician in order to be available to take orders and understand the medical plan of care. If the RN is not able to make rounds with the physician, then the RN must assess the patient's level of understanding the physician. Clarification of the medical plan of care can then be given if necessary. The RN can help write down questions for the patient to refer to when the physician comes by again. If the patient is unable to articulate his or her own needs, then the RN reports the wishes or questions to the physician.

The RN is responsible for assessing the patient's understanding of the plan of care and ensuring that the patient has all the information needed to make informed decisions. An informed patient is empowered to make choices that best meet his or her needs. The RN must be certain that the patient understands the implications of every decision. Furthermore, the RN is in a better position to advocate for the patient who understands the plan of care.

The RN must be a caring individual to be a patient advocate. Caring implies that the RN has a commitment to preserving the patient's humanity, personal worth, and dignity. The patient's humanity is the part that makes him or her unique. It is a mixture of culture, beliefs, spirituality, thoughts, and feelings. The patient who has an acute, chronic, or terminal illness is facing many challenges. The RN demonstrates a caring nature through actions and words that encourage the patient toward holistic wellness. This means that the RN takes an interest in the patient's concerns, establishes dialogue for understanding, and develops a plan of care to meet these needs. Caring means the RN accepts responsibility for providing the best possible care.

Medical Plan of Care

Part of the RN role of advocating for the patient is directing the medical plan of care, but the physician is the manager of the medical plan of care. Medical management of patient care is influenced by an increasing amount of state and federal regulations that restrict payments and limit the number of reimbursable hospital days. For example, physicians must manage care within diagnosis-related group (DRG) designations that set the amount of payment for each medical diagnosis and procedure.

The physician, as medical manager of care, trusts that the plan is implemented in an efficient and effective manner. The RN must anticipate the medical direction, understand the orders written, and foresee how they will affect the patient and patient care (Exercise 13-2). Understanding how a patient responds to the illness as well as to the treatment plan is essential to designing an individualized plan of care. It will also ensure that diagnostic procedures, medications, and treatments ordered by the physician are carried out efficiently and safely. The RN is acting as a patient advocate when making sure that the physician's orders are carried out in a timely fashion. The RN must not cause a delay in diagnosis or treatment based on an incorrect schedule. Equally important is to ensure that the patient's response to one treatment or diagnostic test will not interfere with recovery. Recognizing the adverse affects that may occur at certain times, the RN can take measures to minimize or eliminate them.

More than one physician may be managing different medical problems for one patient. The RN must understand each of these roles and be able

Exercise 13-2

A series of diagnostic radiographs are ordered. The RN must recognize that one has to be done after an enema preparation, another must have the patient NPO, and another might be interfered with by the ingestion of a radiopaque material.

1. What is the priority of care with regard to implementing these orders?

2. If the RN fails to order the diagnostic exams correctly, what could the outcomes be?

to communicate information to whichever physician has a need for it, averting time delays and minimizing physician frustration. Delays in care could place the patient in a compromised position, extend patient care days, and potentially causing harm.

When making a phone call to a physician about a change in patient status, the RN needs to anticipate all the data and information the physician will require to make a decision regarding the medical plan of care. Organizing the data and reporting it in a coherent manner is key to establishing a professional relationship with the physician, not to mention speeding the healing process and positively affecting patient outcomes.

All aspects of patient care require the RN to know how to communicate key information. In collaborative practice the RN is aware of the requirements of each department. Being well organized is important when requesting information, ordering treatments, and communicating with various health care agencies (Exercise 13-3).

The RN must understand the complexities of patient care management in order to advocate for the patient. The RN, either directly or by delegation, must communicate with the physician regarding changes in patient status and priority of care. To advocate in this way, the RN helps the patient receive the best care at the appropriate level and for the least cost. Effective communication includes knowing who is in control of patient discharge or transfer. Generally, the admitting physician is the doctor of record and the one to write discharge orders or to be consulted for transfers. If the patient's problems are related to or compromise the system being managed by the specialist, then this physician will determine the need and write the orders for the change in patient care.

In execution of physician orders, the RN must take into account policies and procedures as well as standing or unit-specific orders. A physician may order medications or treatments that are experimental or not FDA approved for the specific medical disorder of the patient. The RN must be aware of when medications or treatments are being used for anything other than the labeled, intended use. Being a patient advocate means the RN must protect the patient's right to be fully informed. Experimental treatments must have a protocol, and the patient must give informed consent before being included in the treatment plan.

The RN promotes the members of the health care team through understanding and respecting the role, and seeking the expertise, of each. This widens the RN's pool of resources. The RN can call upon a

Exercise 13-3

A patient with end-stage renal disease is being admitted for complications from an imbalance in fluid and electrolytes. The outcome priority is _____ , which includes correcting the fluid overload and electrolyte disturbances. The admitting physician, the patient's nephrologist, has called in an endocrinologist to manage the patient's type II diabetes and an internal medicine physician to rule out a potential stress-related peptic ulcer. The following are the admission orders:

• Chem. 12, and ABGs to be drawn now

• Flat plate abdomen and chest X ray

• Blood cultures × 2

• NG to intermittent suction

The patient has 200 ml of dark red secretions, testing positive for blood, from the NG tube within the first hour. The patient complains of thirst, and the glucometer reading is 260.

1. When the results come back, who will need to have the information?

2. What other questions need to be answered before calling one or both of the physicians?

respiratory therapist with questions regarding the patient's breathing problems and then include the recommended interventions in the plan of care. Working in collaboration with the medical lab, the RN will coordinate the timing of blood draws based on medication, electrolytes, or IV solution.

Discharge Planning

Discharge planning requires the RN to anticipate the needs of the patient beyond the health care facility. More institutions are using discharge planning conferences with discharge specialists, or case managers, who collaborate with the care team to plan for the needs of the patient after discharge. These conferences also address the interventions that will get the patient to the point of discharge in a safe and effective way. The RN's role is to ensure that the right people are involved in the sessions and that needed patient information is available so that the best plan of care can be designed.

Key people in on discharge planning may be physicians, medical social workers, case managers, clinical pharmacists, occupational and physical therapists, respiratory therapist, and pastoral care representative. In institutions that do not have discharge planning sessions, the RN must often communicate the needs of the patient to the physician in order for timely and complete discharge orders to be written.

The RN must be aware of referrals that need to be made within the facility as well as outside the facility. The RN often consults case managers to assist in making referrals to home health agencies, to assisted living units, or for physical or occupational therapy. Knowing the needs of the patient, the RN keeps in communication with the case manager and may even suggest specific referrals. Case managers may work for the institution, for a group of physicians, or for a specific health care plan. Their role is to ensure that the plan of care is being followed within the health care institution and, if needed, continued upon discharge. They assist the hospital and physicians by monitoring the recovery progression and evaluating the priorities of care. They often remind physicians to change the care to serve the patient better. In institutions that do not have case managers, the RN assumes this role of monitoring and assessing the definitive care need.

A patient who leaves an acute care facility before achieving optimum wellness may need continued assistance. Home health agencies can assist a patient in several ways. Knowing the capabilities of the home health referral will assist the RN in coordinating the care of the patient beyond the acute care facility. Agencies are able to provide assistance with basic self-care activities for daily living (ADLs) in the home setting as well as assistance with complex medical treatments. In addition, an increasing number of agencies are able to provide physical therapy, occupational therapy, and respiratory therapy.

The spiritual needs of the patient may be best served by a referral to the pastoral care department, if available. While the RN may have the ability to understand the spiritual needs of the patient, has been trained to use therapeutic communication techniques, and is empathetic to the patient's situation, the pastoral care department specializes in meeting the spiritual needs of the patient. Delegating to the professional with the best resources for meeting the specific needs of the patient improves patient care.

Summary

Being a manager of care is a crucial role for the RN. The patient and the entire health care team have come to rely on the RN for direction and management of minute-to-minute patient care. The manager of care role requires the RN to be a leader with knowledge of the health care team's strengths and weaknesses. The strong leader uses this knowledge to empower the health care team to meet the complex and unique needs of each patient. Collaboration with other health care professionals in carrying out the plan of care is essential, and the nurse is ultimately responsible for coordinating all aspects of patient care within and between the various disciplines. Conflict is inevitable for the manager of care, but the RN can use certain tools to find the optimal resolution. This chapter provided insight into the role of patient advocate, which is also expected of the RN.

Critical Thinking Questions

1. As an RN on a medical-surgical unit, you have a care team that includes two LPNs and a patient care aide. One of the LPNs is a 12-year veteran with IV certification and training to do unit-specific IV pushes. The second LPN has just 2 months' experience, is not IV certified, and has been known to need assistance with complex dressing changes as well as with organizing her day. The patient care aide has 10 years' experience and has had advanced aid training, including in urinary catheter insertion, simple enemas, and advanced

skin care. Assignments and duties for the day include an I&O catheter, an antibiotic IV push, a complex dressing change, an enema prep for a barium, small and large bowel tests, a surgical skin prep, and a patient who will need close supervision due to confusion.

a. What are the safest and most effective patient assignments for each of the team members?

b. Describe the way you would delegate care for a new admission to each of the health care workers who you decide will be able to do the job.

2. An RN must decide not only when to call a physician but what information the physician will need to know. A patient with a history of chronic airway insufficiency has been given a diuretic for fluid retention and slight pulmonary edema. A serum potassium level of 3.2 came back after the diuretic was given.

a. What assessment must be done before notifying the physician?

b. What information must be included when the physician is called regarding the potassium level?

3. Patient assignments have been made, when you overhear an RN state, "I can't believe it: the third day in a row I got this assignment. What does she think she is doing? I get all of the hard assignments, and that Jenny gets all of the easy assignments. Just 2 months out of nursing school, and she gets preferential treatment."

a. How would you respond to this apparent conflict?

b. What may be the basis for the apparent discrepancy in assignments?

c. What information do you need to resolve this conflict?

References

Laschinger HK et al: Leadership behavior impact on staff nurse empowerment, job tension, and work effectiveness, *J Nurs Admin* 29(5):28, 1999.

Marquis BL, Huston CJ: *Leadership roles and management functions in nursing: theory and application,* ed 3, Philadelphia, 2000, Lippincott.

Morrison RS, Jones L, Fuller B: The relation between leadership style and empowerment on job satisfaction of nurses, *J Nurs Admin* 27(5):27, 1997.

Perra BM: The leader in you, *Nurs Manage* 30(1):35, 1999.

Smith S: *Communications in nursing: communicating assertively and responsibly in nursing: a guidebook*, St Louis, 1992, Mosby.

Sullivan EJ, Decker PJ: *Effective management in nursing*, ed 2, Menlo Park, Cal, 1988, Addison-Wesley.

Trofino J: Transformational leadership in health care, *Nurs Manage* 26(8): 42, 1995.

Chapter 14

The RN as a Researcher

Key Terms

active variable
attribute variable
concept
dependent variable
empirical data
experimental design
hypothesis
independent variable
operational definition
performance
  improvement
population

qualitative study
quality assurance
quantitative study
quasi-experimental
  design
reliability
research design
sample selection
sample size
validity
variable

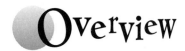

Overview

A growing expectation exists that nursing should become a research-based profession. Utilization of research is a role expectation and standard of care for an RN in the planning and implementation of care for patients. State nursing boards and the Joint Commission on Accreditation for Healthcare Organizations (JCAHO) are more insistent that policies and procedures have a foundation in scientific research. The RN should be able to search the nursing literature to determine whether research findings are available to assist in patient care. Therefore an RN must be able to understand basic research as it applies to the practice as well as practice standards.

This chapter addresses fundamentals of research and research utilization. Components of and steps in the research process are explained. The chapter also gives examples of how research is applied to nursing practice.

Foundation for Research

The RN must recognize the importance of research as it applies to nursing practice and standards of care. The RN should also understand that sound nursing judgement has its basis in scientifically tested rationale. For the RN to utilize research in his or her practice, he or she should have a basic understanding of the investigational process and how it applies to practice. Estabrooks (1999), in conducting a literature search, reports numerous studies that called for nursing to be research based. The author concludes that RNs had difficulty applying research to practice, which is using the scientific process to gain knowledge that has direct application to the practice of nursing or health care. This is not to say that all nurses must conceive of and conduct new research, but certainly all nurses need the ability and the empowerment to appropriately institute change based on research findings. The RN must base specific interventions and all aspects of the nursing process on scientific research.

Apparent Gaps in Research Utilization

Carroll and colleagues (1997) and Mackay (1998) report on the apparent gap in research and research utilization by nurses. Carroll and colleagues

(1997) suggest that nurses have a lack of knowledge as to the availability of research applicable to nursing practice. They also suggest that nurses lack educational preparedness to understand research, which is an apparent barrier to research utilization.

Mackay (1998) has suggested several other barriers to nurses, including lack of support from administration and lack of the authority to institute changes based on research. In some instances, no forum for research-based practice-change proposals to surface and no clear method of launching a trial exist. In an age where most staff nurses are pressed to the limits of time and energy already, incorporating research into practice often falls to the convenience of tradition. This apparent dichotomy with regard to research utilization frustrates the RN faced with decisions about patient care.

Research Both Simple and Necessary

The simplest research the RN will take part in is **quality assurance** (QA), or **performance improvement** (PI), studies, which use data to determine whether patient outcome criteria are being met, charting is complete, or procedures are being done per protocol. The result of these studies is to assist the staff in achieving consistently excellent quality care. Problems in these studies provoke questions that may be answered through the scientific approach.

Components and Process in a Research Study

Research as a discipline has its own methodology and terminology that may seem confusing at first. An RN who has learned to read research critically and understand how it may be applied to the clinical setting will be able to exercise better clinical judgment in planning and implementing the nursing process. Components of a research study, at a basic level, include concepts, variables, and a literature search. From these flow an elementary research process.

Concepts

Basic research is the process of refining a **concept**, which is an abstract idea taken from an observed behavior or characteristic so as to make it usable or applicable. Consider the behavior of a patient exhibiting pain.

The concept is pain, which is defined uniquely by the individual and manifested by the behavior. The pain is an abstraction because another individual cannot experience it in the same way. The concept of pain can be studied as a means to better understand similarities and differences in multiple patients' manifestations of pain. The research attempts to define pain in terms of common behaviors, refining the concept so it can be applied to a population of people rather than just an individual.

Variables

TYPES OF VARIABLES A **variable** is a concept, idea, or attribute that is captured and defined within a research study. Variables are so named because they vary from subject to subject, as with height and weight, propensity to exercise, and personal preferences. Variables are the unique characteristics between one human being and another. Another example of a variable is the environment in which people are, which varies from point to point, from minute to minute, and from day to day. When conducting research, the researcher attempts to control the variables, statistically account for them, or explain them in relationship to what is being studied.

Two types of variables are found in research studies: active and attribute variables. The researcher is attempting to manipulate an **active variable** in an attempt to determine whether this will have the desired effect on the outcome. The researcher has no control over an **attribute variable**. For example, determining the type of dressing most likely to improve patient outcomes would require the RN researcher to study the differences between at least two types of dressings. The dressings would be randomly used on different patients, one group receiving one type and another receiving the second type. The dressings would be the active variable because the researcher is manipulating them. The attribute variables would be the condition of the patients, their sex, and other preexisting characteristics over which the researcher does not have control.

In addition, the researcher makes a distinction between a variable that influences a presumed effect, called the **independent variable**, and a variable that is influenced, called the **dependent variable** (Exercise 14-1). The purpose of the research study is to determine the apparent relationship between the independent variable and the dependent variable. For example, imagine a study looking at length of stay of patients with a certain disorder. The interest is in understanding why patients have varying lengths of stay (dependent variable) and the apparent causative factor (independent variable) for the differences. If the researcher notes a specific problem that seems to cause the increased length of stay, this problem will be designated as an independent variable to see whether an actual relationship exists. The researcher may also spin off further research to see whether the length of stay might be the reason for patients to have specific problems. Here the dependent variable would be the problem the patients are having, and the independent variable would be the length of stay.

DEFINING VARIABLES   In an attempt to control the research as much as possible, the researcher defines the variables. The "tighter" the definitions are, the more precise the research can be. An **operational definition** of a variable specifies the operations associated with collecting the data on that variable, or how the researcher will measure the variable. These operational definitions are expected to be firm so the researcher can formulate a tight research project. The researcher who is going to measure weight as one of the dependent or independent variables must determine whether the weight will be in grams or pounds as well as the type and manufacturer of the scale. The researcher may also need to define when weighing will be conducted, such as a specific time each day or before or after a particular procedure. Thus the variable, weighing time, becomes a unique entity to the particular study and is controlled as much as possible through the operational definition so as to account for discrepancies that might occur.

When the operational definition is too tight, it might interfere with generalizing the research results in practice. For example, a researcher describes a specific instrument that was used to affect an outcome, which is available only for this study. The study supports the usefulness of the instrument to assist the patient to wellness, but because the instrument is not widely available, the findings have little value except to the original researcher.

Literature Search

As part of the conceptualization of the study, the researcher does a literature search to determine whether prior research has been done on the defined problem. The literature search can also identify past research that

Exercise 14-1

Many research studies have related smoking to cancer. Although they do not directly prove that smoking causes cancer, in several studies smoking (independent variable) has been shown to influence lung cancer (dependent variable). In the following examples, what would be the dependent and independent variables?

1. Research is being done to determine whether a relationship exists between the length of time an IV is in the arm and the presence of complications such as phlebitis, infiltration, or pain.

2. A researcher notices that relatives of different patients in an intensive care waiting room tend to know one another's names, answer calls for one another, and ask about the hospitalized member of the family. She wonders whether a relationship exists between the family members' coping abilities and the support that the other unrelated intensive care family members give one another.

3. A research study reports on the increased number of complications and increased intensive care time seen in diabetic patients, versus nondiabetic patients, who have had coronary bypass surgery in which pulmonary artery catheters were used.

can be transferred to the current situation. The literature search can assist in defining the variables, formulating a hypothesis, establishing tools that may be needed to collect data, and clarifying the problem. It may define the theory or identify additional variables that may need to be considered or controlled. The literature search will also suggest areas that are not as well supported by research. Once the research is completed, the literature search serves to support the findings.

Research Process

FYI 14-1 lists the steps in the research process. This section provides a detailed discussion of each step.

Making Predictions

The researcher begins the process of research by making an assumption as to the relationship between the dependent variable and independent variable. Such assumptions are turned into a **hypothesis**, which is a written prediction made by the researcher with regard to the variables. It directs the research by setting limits to the study because the researcher will try to prove or disprove the prediction. Generally, the hypothesis results from a question the researcher has with regard to a specific concept. These questions often come from practice situations where **empirical data**, or objective evidence, would suggest a relationship between the variables. The research is designed to gain as much control as possible to determine whether a relationship exists. The following is an example of a hypothesis:

> Menopausal women who include 40 mg of isolated soy protein in their daily diets report fewer hot flashes and more uninterrupted sleep than those whose diet contains no isolated soy protein.

Defining the Research Study

Research can be approached or conducted in several ways, which are formulated in the **research design**. Research can be either experimental, where the researcher actively participates by introducing an intervention, or nonexperimental, where the researcher observes a situation and collects data without introducing an intervention. **Experimental design** controls the independent variables and randomly assigns the subjects to study

FYI 14-1   **Steps in the Research Process**

1. **Making predictions.** From empirical data within the clinical setting or from reading professional journals, the researcher notices patterns and then makes inferences and hypotheses as to cause and effect or comes up with questions.

2. **Defining the research study.** The researcher outlines how best to ascertain the answers to the questions regarding observations.

3. **Defining the population.** From the questions, the researcher selects who or what can benefit from the research.

4. **Selecting a sample.** The researcher defines a representational model that will reflect the larger population being studied.

5. **Making a data collection plan.** The researcher determines the method by which data will be collected, including the tools, instruments, machines, and research design.

6. **Checking reliability and validity.** The researcher applies certain criteria to test whether instruments, tools, machines, and research designs will give accurate results to the questions or hypothesis being studied.

7. **Collecting data.** The researcher or designated assistants collect data.

8. **Interpreting the results.** With statistical programs that minimize the effects of variables beyond control, the researcher gives meaning to the data that have been collected.

9. **Communicating the results.** The information gained through the research is disseminated to those who can best utilize the findings.

groups. The random assignment helps take care of or explain some of the variables not actually being manipulated by the researchers. **Quasi-experimental design** varies from experimental design in that the researcher does not attempt to randomize the subjects but does attempt to show a relationship between the dependent and independent variables.

Defining the Population

Once the research design is selected, the researcher defines the **population** to be studied. The population chosen is one that will potentially benefit from the study results. For example, the researcher may identify a need for a policy to make an automatic referral to a lactation consultant for all first-time mothers planning on breast-feeding. The researcher believes this will increase the number of successful breast-feeding attempts and would like to design a study to identify the cost-benefit relationship. The population would be defined to include first-time mothers who choose to breast-feed and agree to enter into the study, and exclude mothers who are not first-time mothers. By defining the population in such a way, the researcher attempts to exclude variables that may influence the outcomes, such as previous experience with breast-feeding.

Selecting a Sample

Sample selection is the process of determining a representational model of the entire population on which data can be easily or realistically collected. For example, in a research study regarding the circulatory problems that lead to foot ulcers in diabetics, to look at the entire population of diabetics would be unrealistic. If a cross-section of diabetic patients with various characteristics representative of the entire population could be studied, then the sample would be statistically strong. The **sample size** is determined through statistics that take into account general characteristics of the population in question and give a probability number that will closely account for the varied characteristics within the sample size. The sample size might be 50 or 100 subjects, or it could be a thousand or more subjects, but it needs to be within the resources of the researcher.

In addition, inferences may be made about how the variable relationships can be generalized to subjects not defined within the population. These generalizations tend to suggest areas for further study, which can assist in refining the original hypothesis and making research utilization applicable to greater numbers of subjects within the population.

Making a Data Collection Plan

The researcher develops a plan to collect data that includes the method, the necessary tools, the people designated to collect the data, and any training needed. A **quantitative study** asks the question who, what, why, where, when, or how and attempts to describe the relationship between one variable and another. A quantitative study plan is highly structured and controlled. A **qualitative study** attempts to clarify underlying assumptions that are vague or unclear by asking what the perceptions, beliefs, or tenets are within a particular setting. A qualitative study is loosely structured and allows more subjective input from both the researcher and the subjects. Often qualitative studies generate questions for quantitative study. Among the tools used to collect data are self-reports, surveys, questionnaires, graphs, and unique designs specifically developed to measure a variable.

Generally, the researcher conducts a pilot study to work out unforeseen problems with the main study or the study tools and determine whether the research is feasible. The pilot study may include a small part of the population and may include ways to determine whether the tools are measuring what they are expected to measure or whether any instrument that the researcher uses is impractical.

Checking Reliability and Validity

Reliability and validity are criteria that researchers use to test whether instruments, tools, machines, and research designs will give accurate results with the questions or hypotheses being studied. **Reliability** measures the device or technique, or the instrument, the researcher uses to collect data by asking how trustworthy it is at gathering the intended data. The researcher would not want to use an instrument with low reliability because it would skew the results of the study. The instrument could be a questionnaire, interview technique, observation, test, or machines, monitors, scales, or other devices or methods. Several tests for reliability, stability, consistency, and equivalence exist, and the results are reported as decimals, such as "0.89 internal consistency." An example of a test for reliability would be to use an external monitor to record venous oxygen saturation. If the external monitor consistently recorded venous oxygen saturation within 1% or 2% of venous blood draws or another machine with a proven record of reliability, then the research instrument would have a high degree of reliability.

Validity measures the degree to which an instrument is measuring what it is supposed to measure. Validity has various aspects, such as content validity, criterion-related validity, and construct validity. Validity can be difficult to measure with accuracy, and the researcher may settle for a specific level of validity. For example, a researcher may be testing whether a correlation exists between the APGAR scores of newborns and tachypnea of newborns. The researcher will document the tested validity report of the APGAR scoring instrument as an indication of the validity of the new study. Consistency in how the APGAR score is assigned must also be considered as part of the validity study.

Collecting Data

Once the sample has been defined and selected and the instrument proposed, the process of collecting data begins. Data collection within an institution needs to be approved by the research review committee of the health care organization. A research report will include the approval of the committee as well as any patient consent forms that may be needed. Ethical and legal issues raised by the research must be considered and addressed before the actual collection of the data. A research report generally mentions the ways subject rights were protected.

Interpreting the Results

Once the data have been collected, the researcher interprets the results, which requires providing information on how the data were analyzed, what limitations were identified, and how the results support the hypothesis. A formal statistical analysis is able to assist the researchers in demonstrating how close the data came to demonstrating a statistically significant relationship between the variables. In addition, the results are examined for how they may apply to the larger population as well as the study population. Often further research questions are asked due to the outcomes or to limitations that are discovered.

Communicating the Results

Communicating the results so nurses will be able to use the findings in their practice is the final step. Research summaries may be submitted for publication, including a section that demonstrates how the research will apply to nursing. This application may be implied, or it may be stated clearly. If implied, the interpretation of the results will need to be made by the reader of the research article. The use of the information by the RN will require thoughtful consideration.

Research Utilization

The RN is expected to follow certain policies and procedures when acting as a manager of care. The standard of care expectation is that these policies and procedures be based on scientific research. The RN should recognize situations in which clinical judgment might be required, and in such situations research-based decisions will have better outcomes than decisions based on tradition. The RN should also be aware of how research can affect the nursing process, requiring the RN to read research articles critically. The RN can take a research course, attend continuing education classes on research, or read research textbooks to better understand the research process. Utilization of research does not necessarily require the RN to be proficient at conducting research. It does require RNs to make a sound judgment as to the reliability and validity of the research, and ultimately make the decision as to whether to include the findings in one's practice.

Validating Research Results

Some basic steps should be followed in order to identify whether a research report is valid and can be used to make a change in thinking or support a clinical judgment regarding patient care. The first step is to understand the terminology of research. Familiarization with the definitions and examples allow the RN to read the research articles with more understanding. The second step is to conduct a literature search, identifying other research that has been done in the problem area. Ovid and Medline provide access to nursing and allied health journals. Medical libraries within hospitals as well as medical universities have online access to both Ovid and Medline.

Actual research reports contain all components of the research, reporting on the problem, variables, research design, population, and sample, as well as results, discussion, and the application to practice. A journal article may report on original research or on literature search findings. Articles reporting on literature searches do not give complete pictures of each research study but rather summarize the results of several studies. The RN should read the original research reports to decide whether the interpretations are accurate or useful. Generally, articles accepted by nursing or allied health journals that have a peer review or juried acceptance process will have credible research. Even so, the RN should still critically read in order to determine whether the research has applications to practice.

Applying Research to Practice

After reading research, the RN should put into practice what he or she has learned. Eastabrooks (1999) suggests that an RN in the practice setting can utilize research in three main ways:

1. *Direct research utilization* is the use of research knowledge to actually change a practice habit or include a new intervention in your practice. Direct utilization of research by the RN would constitute a personal commitment to change for the betterment of the practice. The RN would actively and critically read research to find new ways to implement patient care that is safer and promotes positive patient outcomes. An example would be to find research on a particular nursing intervention, such as a new technique to start IVs in children that reduces pain and gains more trust. The RN who begins to use the intervention has directly utilized research to effect a change in practice.

2. *Indirect research utilization* is when the RN has a new conceptual understanding of situations or treatments based on knowledge of current research. Enhancing the knowledge base is a direct result of indirect research utilization. If the RN is able to identify a new patient problem as a result of reading a research article, theRN is utilizing research to enhance assessment of the patient's response to the illness or treatment. The greater knowledge gained by the scientific approach has increased the RN's critical thinking abilities and should create positive outcomes as a result. The RN should be better able to plan patient care with clear rationales.

3. *Persuasive research utilization* is the process of advocating for a change in policy or procedure, behavioral change of an individual, or a change in the way things are normally done, based on research awareness. For example, working on a committee that is updating policies and procedures, the RN may advocate a specific policy change based on research.

The RN must recognize the need to read and incorporate research into practice, which is becoming a practice standard. The RN should follow and understand policies and procedures but also know that even policies and procedures must be research based. If the RN is aware of policies and procedures that are not current to practice standards, then it is time to advocate change. The RN can begin by giving the unit manager a written report summarizing the research findings and including a proposal for change. The RN can also propose to run a research study that will demonstrate the benefits of the change in policy. In this way the staff RN can play an important role in developing research.

Read the scenario in Exercise 14-2 and answer the questions concerning the three ways to utilize research.

Identifying Areas for Research

The staff nurse is aware of empirical data (objective evidence from clinical observations) gathered from patient care experiences. Such experiences are often the basis for research questions. Staff RNs may be recruited to take part in the study through data gathering or testing new procedures or products. Encouraging all nurses to bring research into their daily practice will ultimately help improve patient care.

Summary

Research utilization is a practice standard, and the RN who knows how to read and interpret research will gain the knowledge needed to make better clinical judgments. Striving for excellence in nursing is a worthy goal, and gaining knowledge is one way to attain excellence. The RN must have a basic foundation in research utilization to best meet the needs of patients. Knowledge that has its foundation in scientific study will assist the RN in making optimal clinical judgments as well as formulating a sound plan of care.

Exercise 14-2

On a particular medical-surgical floor, many patients are being admitted who have decubitis ulcers, also known as pressure ulcers. The risk factors for developing pressure ulcers have been widely studied and disseminated in literature as well as in educational arenas.

In admission assessments the RN decides to begin including assessing for pressure ulcer risk factors in each of the patients admitted to the unit. If the RN compiled assessment data that supported the research findings on risk factors for decubitus ulcer formation, it will also lend credence to the RN's original clinical judgment. Critical thinking skills are improved, and the RN is better able to plan care that meets the holistic needs of the patient. The RN then takes the information gathered during the assessment of several patients at risk for decubitus ulcers, along with research findings in the literature, and persuades management to change the admission forms to include a standard decubitus ulcer risk assessment.

1. In this scenario, which would be direct, indirect, and persuasive uses of research?

2. Give another example of direct, indirect, and persuasive uses of research that you would utilize within your practice.

Critical Thinking Questions

1. A traditional nursing intervention has been to conduct daily weights on patients between the hours of 4:00 and 6:00 AM.

   a. If the nursing staff notices that patients with ordered daily weights showed less satisfaction compared with patients who did not have daily weights, what questions would need to be asked with regard to the relationship between the time of the daily weights and patient satisfaction?

   b. Conduct a literature search to see whether any research studies are related to the time of day when weights must be done; patient satisfaction and the traditional time for daily weights; and nurses' perceptions of the need for weights at a specific time.

2. Pick a policy or procedure in a health care agency and note whether research citations exist within its rationale statement. If no citation exists, conduct a literature search of research that would either support the policy or procedure or suggest the need for change. How would this information affect the standard of care as interpreted within the policy or procedure?

3. Medication A is ordered to be given to a pediatric patient with an acute asthma attack. The physician has ordered the dose to be 250 mg q6h around the clock. The recommended dosage for pediatric patients is to receive 50 mg/kg/24 hr in divided doses qid.

   a. For a patient who weighs 30 lb, what is the recommended dose?

   b. Is the ordered dose within safe limits?

   c. What type of research utilization would be best for advocating for a patient with a physician who consistantly ignores recommended medication doses?

   d. How would you communicate your findings to the physician in a professional manner?

References

Carroll DL et al: Barriers and facilitators to the utilization of nursing research, *Clin Nurs Spec* 11(5):207, 1997.

Estabrooks CA: The conceptual structure of research utilization, *Res Nurs Health* 22(3):203, 1999.

Mackay MH: Research utilization and the CNS: confronting the issues, *Clin Nurs Spec* 12(6):232, 1998.

Section 5

Role Differences in Managing the Consumer: The Health-Illness Continuum

Chapter 15

Primary Health Care: Factors Influencing Health Promotion

Key Terms

developmental need
health-deviation need
health-illness continuum
Health Promotion
  Matrix
physical environment

primary health care
self-care ability
self-care deficit
self-care requisite
self-health promotion
universal need

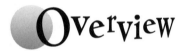

Overview

Primary health care establishes an environment conducive to a healthy lifestyle. Interventions that promote a healthy lifestyle include health screening, immunization, teaching, and role modeling (of a healthy lifestyle). To develop individualized plans of care based on health promotion, you will need to have an understanding of environmental factors that influence health promotion within society and with your individual patients.

This chapter addresses primary health care within a theoretical framework. Included are basic tools that will assist you in understanding your role in health promotion and a discussion of the relationship between your own health and the ability to affect your patients' self-health behaviors.

Theoretical Framework

Every person moves along a **health-illness continuum,** between states of illness and wellness, throughout life, as well as between independence of and dependence on health care services (Figure 15-1). During times of illness, a person seeks assistance from health care services. The initial level of need can be minimal to nearly complete dependence, but the patient will gain the knowledge and skills necessary to regain independence. **Primary health care** promotes independence and involves many interventions, with the goal of maintaining independent, healthy individuals in a community.

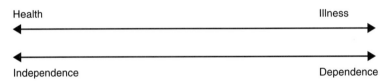

Figure 15-1 Health-illness continuum.

Self-Care

Orem (2001) believes that every individual has some **self-care ability**, which is the day-to-day personal care needed to function and develop. This ability is affected by several things, including but not limited to the individual's age, developmental stage, health, and environmental factors.

Orem (2001) states that the goal for all adults is to have the power and capability to care for themselves. Adults seek assistance when they have a **self-care deficit**, having needs that go beyond their resources to manage. They seek nursing care because of the specific knowledge nurses have and because of their ability to act in association with other health care professionals to assist the patient in regaining self-care ability. Health promotion deals with "what is known about (1) human structure and functioning and (2) specific diseases or interferences with the normal human condition" (p.130). Orem assumes that the responsibility of primary health promotion is with the individual adult. Within the realm of health promotion, someone may seek a higher level of function or development, thus seeking out nurses who have special knowledge of ways to achieve this goal. Nurses are involved in health promotion when the following take place:

1. People are under the direct care of a nurse.
2. The nurse is engaging in practices that prevent or interrupt the disease process, in the environment of the patient.
3. The nurse is guiding people toward health prevention methods.
4. The nurse is incorporating factual information about the patient into the plan of care.
5. The nurse is aware that the adult or responsible adult will be the primary person to carry out the plan of care.

In terms of health promotion, the nurse's role is working with people with generally good health but who are experiencing life or development changes. Health promotion efforts by nurses are educational efforts to help the individual remain an independent self-care agent (Figure 15-2).

Global Health Promotion

Gorin and Arnold (1998) present health promotion as a multidimensional effort by numerous agencies and individuals at the global, national, and local levels. Health promotion has both individual and social contexts.

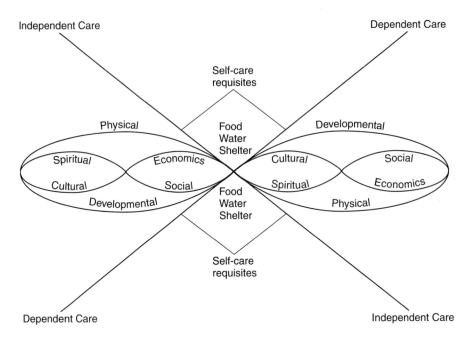

Figure 15-2 Environmental influence on health promotion.

It includes both diverse and complementary approaches to effecting posi-tive health behaviors. Health promotion can directly eliminate hazards or threats to health, as in the efforts of the Environmental Protection Agency, or be indirect, such as educational programs that present lifestyle changes and inoculation programs that hope to decrease the incidence of disease. Nurses work with government and private, nonprofit, and community agencies in the delivery of health promotion services.

Health Promotion Model

Pender and Pender (1996) present a revised Health Promotion Model that makes specific assertions with regard to health promotion. Key to the model are characteristics and experiences as influenced by the individual's perceptions, as well as the interpersonal and situational influences on health. Pender and Pender do not state that a clear association exists between any one influence and the healthy behavior outcomes, including individual commitment to health-promoting behaviors. An example is the differences in two individuals' responses to a broken leg. One sees an opportunity to take time off from work, is challenged to figure out how to complete ADLs, and is looking forward to catching up on reading. The other finds the experience to be limiting, gets angry when not able to do something easily or when needing help with ADLs, and gets bored not being able to go to work. The first person is easygoing, takes day-to-day challenges in stride, and has no problem seeking assistance when situations warrant. The second finds working pleasurable at the expense of recreation and has trouble delegating or seeking consultation from fellow workers or friends. Pender and Pender (1996) infer that every factor has some degree of influence on healthy behaviors, and consideration of these will need to take place for the nurse to know how to assist these patients.

The nurse should engage in health-protective behaviors as well as health promotion behaviors. Health protective behaviors take a person away from a dangerous situation or from a dangerous habit. Deciding not to smoke, not going near a burning building, and not crossing the street except at designated crosswalks all protect one's health. Health promotion behaviors move an individual to a higher level of health, greater vigor, or energy to do more than he or she is currently capable.

Self-Health Promotion

As an LPN, maintaining a healthy lifestyle is important. Remaining healthy will optimize your transition through school to become an RN. A healthy lifestyle also bolsters self-confidence, which is even more important as you assume the responsibilities of an RN. Furthermore, to promote healthy lifestyles in your patients, you first must model a healthy lifestyle. As RNs, you need to practice what you preach. It would be difficult to help a patient stop smoking if you were to smoke. Modeling a healthy lifestyle empowers others to emulate the good habits, especially if we share our stories along the way. **Self-health promotion** also lends credibility to your role as patient advocate.

Health Promotion Principles

Gorin and Arnold (1998) envision a **Health Promotion Matrix** as a clinical tool for the RN. This model recognizes that the individual is surrounded by and influenced by client systems of family, group, and community. These systems can have a positive, supportive influence or a negative influence on the client's health promotion. These systems formulate the client's image and image processing of his or her health, health behaviors, and ability to seek help for them. Thus a family of smokers and perhaps several peer smokers may influence an individual who is a smoker. Their perceptions or images of their health behavior and willingness to stop smoking may be strongly influenced by the systems. If the family is a nonsupportive system, the members not supporting the cessation efforts of the individual, then the attempt to successfully quit smoking will be compromised. Your role as an RN in this situation may be to gather other support systems, such as smoking cessation support groups, in order to optimize the individual's chances of cessation success.

Orem (2001) considers self-care as meeting one's own basic needs, including the self-care requisites of universal, developmental, and health-deviation needs. A **universal need** is an essential requirement for everyone: food, shelter, air, water, and other basic needs. A **developmental need**, such as trust, love, and belonging, changes as a person moves through each life-cycle period. A **health-deviation need** is based on an individual's genetic or constitutional deviations from normal.

Orem recognizes that to meet self-care requisites, a person must have knowledge of the self-care requisite need. A **self-care requisite** could be a universal need, an essential that everyone must have to sustain and nurture life. Such needs are basic to human life (food, water, rest, and so on) as well as specific cultural, social, environmental, and enrichment requirements that the individual deems necessary for growth and development. Individuals also need a supportive environment, and they must be willing to engage in internal and external orientation activities that promote health. Thus an individual may engage in a weight reduction program in which he or she may meet once a week with others to be supported in his or her effort (external orientation). This individual may also engage in reading self-help books to discover ways to rid himself or herself of negative feelings that promote the unhealthy eating habits (internal orientation). A person must also be willing and able to access available resources to meet the self-care requisite needs (FYI 15-1).

The importance of external and internal influences on a person's health promotion is evident, and we must assess these influences to begin the health-promotion plan of care. A holistic assessment process takes into consideration all factors that assist in or inhibit meeting goals.

FYI 15-1   Self-Care Requisites

To meet self-care requisites, the RN does the following:

- Identifies potential and actual social support systems
- Understands the patient's point of view
- Considers the developmental task
- Understands the patient's self-care abilities

Health Promotion Plan of Care

A health promotion plan of care includes education and self-actualization exercises to help the individual seek a higher level of health (Figure 15-3). For example, someone may need to gain an understanding of why he or she is overweight before getting involved in a weight-reduction program. The plan of care should allow the person time to come to terms with the basis of the weight problem. The comprehensive health care plan reflects all health concerns, rather than focusing on just weight reduction, so the RN in this case needs to assess for such weight-related problems as hypertension, hyperlipidemia, and diabetes as well. A holistic plan of care takes into account the total person and how all his or her characteristics influence outcomes.

The priority of care for health promotion is to help a patient or client regain control over his or her health. The priority nursing diagnoses include health-seeking behaviors or knowledge deficit. Outcome criteria and the measurement of outcomes focus on the progress toward the primary goal of a higher level of health. The patient will need to be included in planning the care as a means to empowerment and compliance.

The RN's Role in Health Promotion

Besides designing individual plans of care, the RN can also be proactive in health promotion on a local or regional political level. One way to

Assessment: Assess individual or group:

1. Level of wellness

    a. What are the individual or group self-care abilities?

    b. What factors are interfering in the maintenance of a wellness state (e.g., smoking, high cholesterol level, poor sleep habits, stress)?

2. Readiness to change to a higher state of health

    a. What is the motivation to change?

    b. What will actually or potentially interfere with change?

    c. Is the environment suitable for learning?

3. Understanding self-care needs

    a. What cultural, spiritual, and social needs exist?

    b. What language and educational needs exist?

    c. What limitations of sight, hearing, or speech exist?

    d. What self-care limitations exist?

4. Understanding self-care knowledge

    a. What information does the individual or group have?

    b. What myths, assumptions, or inferences exist?

    c. What questions are being presented?

    d. What concerns are being voiced?

Outcome identification: Voiced satisfaction of level of understanding, compliance with wellness plan of care, specific measurable criteria related to individualized plan of care (e.g., weight loss, cholesterol levels lowered, blood pressure under control).

Planning: Decide whether the following exist:

1. A knowledge deficit related to at-risk behaviors, noncompliance with healthy lifestyle.

2. Health seeking behavior related to new diagnosis/treatment and/or voicing of concerns with current treatment plan, voiced need to change life to a healthy lifestyle.

Implementation: Support of self-care ability:

1. Provide education at an individual level of understanding, using a preferred learning style.

2. Assist the individual or group in setting a schedule or plan with clear, measurable goals.

3. Reinforce progress.

4. Help client cope with disappointments or setbacks; be available for venting of frustrations.

5. Use support groups or individual counseling as a means to share difficulties and progress.

6. Provide information on classes or other avenues (e.g., the Internet) for further education.

7. Individualize tools for reminders if there is a need for scheduled events (e.g., handmade calendars, refrigerator magnet reminders, 7-day pill dispensers); be creative and incorporate the individual's suggestions.

Evaluation: Evaluate effectiveness:

1. Stick to set time frames for evaluating progress.

2. Use outcome criteria as a basis for evaluation.

3. Assess patient satisfaction for progress toward a higher level of wellness.

Figure 15-3 Health promotion plan of care.

become politically involved is to provide expert testimony to governing bodies in an attempt to promote a more positive health environment. For example, a nurse can testify on the effects of environmental pollution on the health of a community or lobby through letters to representatives, advocating changes in legislation with regard to pollution. On a local level, the RN can offer services to church groups, PTAs, or neighborhood organizations as educators or by assisting with public awareness of problems identified within the community. As RNs, we recognize the importance of research as a way to identify cause-and-effect situations and support or provide interventions to make a change. If we actively engage in health promotion, we will be of value to the communities in which we live.

Environmental Influences on Health Promotion

Everyone exists within an environment, the surroundings or conditions that exert an influence on, and affect the health of, a person. One's environment is made up of physical, cultural, spiritual, social, economic, and developmental components (FYI 15-2). The environment can be supportive of a healthy lifestyle, or it can be a source of stress. The RN must recognize the influence of the environment on people's health care abilities.

FYI 15-2   Environments That Influence Health Promotion

- Physical
- Cultural
- Spiritual or religious
- Social
- Economic
- Developmental

Physical

The **physical environment** is composed of tangible factors where the individual lives, from housing, furniture, and food to pollution, air, temperature, and bacteria. Physical factors have concrete characteristics that can be seen, felt, tasted, touched, or measured in some way.

The degree to which the physical environment influences the individual can generally be detected through direct measurement. For example, air pollution has been studied in relationship to many respiratory conditions. Many research studies show that individuals with asthma have more acute attacks when higher pollen counts or high smog numbers are present. Community public health departments often lead such studies and will make recommendations or issue public announcements warning of the increased risks during periods of air-quality problems. Another example, with perhaps longer-term consequences, is the relationship between high levels of lead in public housing and the number of health problems suffered by children living in this environment.

Health promotion related to the physical environment begins with assessment of the characteristics of the environment that have been implicated as causing health variations for the individual or the community. A plan of care is developed to minimize the negative influence of the physical environment (Exercise 15-1). Interventions focus on either avoidance of the environmental factors or modifying lifestyles to minimize their effects.

Patient satisfaction with modifications in lifestyle will be an important component in evaluating any plan of care that attempts to change behavior to minimize environmental influence. For example, an individual with great affection for pets may also be allergic to them. The obvious solution, avoiding pets, may not be an acceptable intervention. A creative approach will be needed to minimize the person's response to the allergens while including the pets in the life plan. The pet owner may still have an acceptable level of allergic response, which will be part of the individual's definition of health. The RN must accept such client decisions, while promoting a healthier lifestyle.

Cultural, Spiritual, and Social

The cultural, spiritual, and social components of the environment play a major role in how an individual views health and illness. One's personal

Exercise 15-1

An individual is diagnosed with asthmatic allergies, where cedar pollen has been identified as one of the allergic triggers for asthma events. In planning interventions, the nurse should know that airborne allergens are difficult to avoid.

1. How could the plan incorporate measures to minimize exposure to cedar pollen?

2. What interventions would not only minimize the effects of the allergens but also support the patient's need to remain independent?

beliefs are generally formed as he or she grows up. As part of the community, the RN is in a position to understand how these individual beliefs can influence the general health of the community as well as the health of the individual. By being able to evaluate these environmental influences, the nurse can begin to formulate a list of potential health risks and actual problems.

Cultural influences on health are most obviously observed in the form of dietary habits. For example, as a whole, Americans consume a higher degree of fat and empty calories in their diet than other cultures. As a result, a large percentage of the United States population develops negative health consequences, such as peripheral vascular disease, coronary artery disease, hypertension, obesity, and diabetes. Culture may have a more subtle influence on the way individuals seek health care. In some cultures, people are not encouraged to seek help. The RN should recognize cultural influences that will bias the health-seeking behaviors of individuals because this information will help define the needs of each person within a community.

Spiritual or religious support for health promotion may come from a person's perception of help from a higher power (Gorin and Arnold, 1998). This may manifest itself in practices, dictated by a religious body's beliefs, that are geared to promote spiritual as well as physical health, such as prayer for health and rituals believed to be health promoting. Additionally, many spiritual practices, such as therapeutic touch and spiritualism, are engaged in to regain health or restore spiritual well-being. The RN has the opportunity to encourage or support spiritual activities that promote an individual's health (Exercise 15-2).

Social support can come from immediate family members, friends, employers and co-workers, neighbors, the community (e.g., community

Exercise 15-2

Religion plays an important role in health-seeking behaviors and in health promotion. For example, your patient's religious beliefs forbid the use of vaccines.

1. What would a health promotion plan of care look like?

2. Without trying to change the individual's beliefs, how would you as RN in the educator role encourage a healthier lifestyle?

centers), and state and national agencies (e.g., Red Cross, United Way, Social Security Administration, and U.S. Department of Health and Human Services). People who are gainfully employed and able to provide for their own basic needs may access social support to help them cope with life stresses. People who are not as fortunate may access local or federal agencies for support for basic needs as well as for coping with life stresses. Everyone defines the support that he or she needs.

Systems of support are frameworks developed by the individual to assist in networking within the community. The two basic systems of support are closed and open systems. Someone with a closed system seeks support within the immediate or defined family. Someone with an open system looks beyond the family for sources of support. Most people move along the continuum from closed to open system as needs dictate. Healthy individuals generally have a balance of internal and external support systems.

Economic

The economic environment may influence health-seeking behavior. Low-income families generally access the health care system for preventive care less frequently than families with moderate to upper levels of income. Additionally, it is more likely that women and children of low socioeconomic status will not be insured (Drevdahl, 1999; Johnson, 2001; Polivka et al, 2000; Swider, 2002).

Many health promotion options are available for low-income families and individuals. Public health and private, nonprofit organizations provide many low-cost or essentially free services. Well-baby and women's health clinics are public, subsidized health promotion sites for low income individuals. Private-practice wellness clinics and "fast-track" clinics are now emerging as replacements for, or alternatives to, public health programs. The incentive of these emerging clinics is to provide medical assistance directly to infants, children, and families, and they establish a system of care that minimizes the need to use emergency rooms for minor or nonemergent health concerns.

The economic health of a community affects the primary health care offering. If the economy is not strong, an agency that could otherwise support the community will not have the resources to meet preventive health needs. For example, smoking cessation classes and well-baby clinics that focus on illness prevention will be sacrificed for the community's more universal infrastructure needs, such as roads and sanitation.

Establishing continuity of care in populations that traditionally place a burden on community resources provides the community with a cost benefit. However, barriers may still exist that prevent access to these health promotion sites. Transportation to and from the clinics can be cost prohibitive to people unable to afford their own transportation and without access to public transportation.

Perception of potential or actual economic consequences to one's wellness state can influence health-seeking behavior. If the cost of improving health or maintaining a current level of health is perceived as being greater than the individual can manage, then the healthy behaviors may be ignored. For example, even if an individual understands that he or she needs to take antilipid medication prescribed by the physician, without insurance or financial resources it is unlikely that he or she will continue the medication or even fill the prescription in the first place. Low-income families may not have enough money to afford even reduced copayments for preventive medications, much less maintain a supply of healthy foods.

Church and other nonprofit organizations may become invaluable partners for an RN formulating a plan of care. Matching the resources of community organizations with people in need is part of coordinating a far-reaching health plan. An RN can thus be a catalyst for change in the overall health of the neighborhood, town, state, and nation.

Developmental

Age-related and developmental factors also affect health-seeking behaviors. Development theorists attempt to define the process of physical and psychosocial growth as being predictable and orderly (Taylor, Lillis, and LeMone, 2001). Development has many influences, including heredity, temperament, and emotion, as well as the physical, psychological, and social environments. Eric Erickson is probably the most influential developmental theorist relative to nursing. His theory bases psychosocial development on the process of socialization, or how people interact with and react to the world. Erickson recognized the influences of social interactions, the environment, and biology on the eight stages of life. Each person moves from or stays at a developmental level as a result of resolution of conflicts there (Potter and Perry, 2001; Taylor, Lillis, and LeMone, 2001). See FYI 15-3 for Erickson's 8 stages of development.

Fundamental concepts of development theory include adaptive potential; that adaptive abilities derive in part from cultural, hereditary, and

FYI 15-3 **Erickson's 8 Stages of Development**

Stage	Associated Task
Infancy	Trust versus mistrust
Toddler	Autonomy versus shame
Early childhood	Initiative versus guilt
Middle childhood	Industry versus inferiority
Adolescence	Identity versus identity diffusion
Adulthood	Intimacy versus isolation
Middle age	Generativity versus self-absorption
Old age	Integrity versus despair

environmental influences; and that each person strives for self-actualization within his or her world (Potter and Perry, 2001). *Self-actualization* is an individual's understanding of his or her abilities and roles within a culture, community, society, or world.

These developmental concepts describe positive or negative influences on health-seeking behaviors or compliance with a health promotion plan of care. For example, a 40-year-old man may be working to provide for a growing family and plan for a future retirement. Health promotion may be on his mind, but he may be caught up in self-imposed time constraints that may make it difficult to maintain a healthy lifestyle and may not perceive that he has the time or energy to take up the task of self-health promotion. The RN must understand this individual's developmental tasks and view before developing a trusting relationship. Trust is needed to develop a collaborative plan that takes into consideration the individual's need to maintain current life goals as much as possible.

Development progresses in an orderly fashion throughout the life span. Each individual progresses at his or her own rate, which means that some people's developmental levels may not correlate with age expectations. For example, a 50-year-old man who engages in drag racing on public streets or in unsafe sexual practices is modeling the high-risk behavior more typical of the developmental stage of early adulthood or late adolescence. The RN, in collaborating with this person on a health promotion plan of care, may come to realize that what this man considers important may actually interfere with his ability to understand the relationship of health promotion and decreasing high-risk behavior. The health promotion plan of care needs to include an exploration of why he continues to engage in high-risk behavior before interventions can be implemented to assist in changing the behavior.

Many factors influence the developmental age of the individual and can influence the response to health-seeking behaviors. Individuals under stress tend to rely on successful adaptive measures learned in the past, behaviors that may be health promoting or in fact detracting from health. For example, a woman who quit smoking 5 years ago is now facing the possibility of a divorce. This life change has great significance and a high degree of stress. Remembering the times when she would smoke to calm herself when she was feeling anxious, the woman decides to start smoking again. A health promotion plan of care must focus on redirecting the unhealthy attempt to cope with healthier alternatives, such as support groups, counseling, or other positive-diversion activities.

Nursing diagnoses for developmental plans of care include "Health-seeking behaviors," "High risk for ineffective coping, individual/family," and "Knowledge deficit." The priority of care is to maintain an environment that is optimal for growth and development. Outcome criteria are individualized but should include indicators that developmental milestones are being met and that the person is maintaining a healthy lifestyle and is satisfied with the progress being made. The RN who is willing to collaborate with the individual can design a strong health promotion plan of care.

Primary Health Care Systems

While health promotion is a portion of the nurse's role, many other organizations and individuals provide primary health care. The family nurse practitioner and the family practice physician are primary health care providers. Patients seek them out and trust that their counsel will help keep them well. The primary services they provide include physicals, immunizations, screening for potential health problems, and monitoring health and well-being. The RN can refer to the family practice physician or the nurse practitioner as part of the health promotion plan of care.

Public health is another area with a focus on health promotion. Generally, public health promotion centers on a framework of public policies that dictate the economic and bureaucratic structure of the agencies. From the World Health Organization to the state and local health departments, the main focus is setting standards for health, implementing interventions to meet the standards, and monitoring the outcomes in an effort to improve the general health of the community. Constraints and benefits are often linked to an agency's ability to maintain the intended level of health promotion. On a national level, legislative regulations, budgetary concerns, and patients' rights can dictate the effectiveness of the programs. Federal and state regulations focus on actions that minimize potentially widespread health problems. Programs of vaccination, preschool health screening, reporting of specific diseases, and gathering of health statistics minimize the influence of potential or actual health concerns.

Summary

On an individual patient basis, the RN recognizes that many extenuating environmental circumstances can interfere with a healthy lifestyle and with health promotion efforts. Innumerable global and local factors affect the health of the individual as well as that of the collective population. The RN is in a position to take a lead in health promotion through role-modeling a healthy lifestyle. In collaboration with other health care team members, the RN can design a plan of care with consideration of the needs and influences of the individual, family, and community. The goal of health promotion efforts is a higher level of function and development to allow the patient or client independence and empowerment to make healthy life choices.

Critical Thinking Questions

1. Working at a health fair, you screen a participant who presents with a blood pressure reading of 190/110 mm Hg. By talking with her, you find that she

has a history of hypertension, but she does not like to take pills. "My mother kept us well without medications, and when she died, she was on at least 10 different medications. I just don't trust a system that hands out pills for every little thing."

a. What questions would you ask of this person?

b. What is the definitive care priority that is related to the health promotion or prevention need?

2. A minister at your church approaches you to give a talk at a Tuesday Family Night gathering. You would like to do a health promotion talk but are unsure of the best topic.

a. What assessment questions would you formulate to identify an important health promotion need?

b. What potential health concern would a person who was raised within a Catholic, Jewish, Protestant, American Indian, Mexican American, or other subculture have?

c. What would be the health promotion care priority for this cultural health concern?

3. The physician has ordered a weight reduction diet for an overweight individual with high cholesterol. The physician does not want the patient to have more than 20% fat in his diet.

a. Of an 1800-calorie diet, how many calories should be in fat?

b. What would a typical day's balanced menu look like, when the approximate weight or portion size of each of the items has been taken into account?

References

Drevdahl D: Meanings of community in a community health center, *Public Health Nurs* 16(6):417, 1999.

Gorin SS, Arnold J: *Health promotion handbook,* St Louis, 1998, Mosby.

Johnson MO: Meeting health care needs of a vulnerable population: perceived barriers, *J Community Health Nurs* 18(1):35, 2001.

Orem DE: *Nursing concepts of practice,* ed 6, St Louis, 2001, Mosby.

Pender NJ, Pender AR: *Health promotion in nursing practice,* ed 3, Norwalk, Conn, 1996, Appleton & Lange.

Polivka BJ et al: Hospital and emergency department use by young low-income children, *Nurs Res* 49(5):253, 2000.

Potter P, Perry A: *Fundamentals of nursing,* ed 5, St Louis, 2001, Mosby.

Swider SM: Outcome effectiveness of community health workers: an integrative literature review, *Public Health Nurs* 19(1):11, 2002.

Taylor C, Lillis C, LeMone P: *Fundamentals of nursing: the art and science of nursing,* ed 4, Philadelphia, 2001, Lippincott.

Chapter 16

Managing Care in Secondary and Tertiary Health Care

Key Terms

clinical pathway
consequence
cultural strain
dependent-care agency
manager of care
secondary (acute) health
 care
self-care agency
social support
spiritual distress
tertiary care

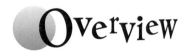

Overview

A person enters the acute health care setting when he or she is without sufficient resources for self-care and in need of the specialized skills of the nurse to meet the dependent care needs brought on by the illness. To varying degrees, the individual who enters the acute care setting enters into a collaborative relationship with the health care team. The realm of the RN, nursing, is managing care related to the patient's response to the acute illness state, the pharmacological interventions, and the surgical and medical plan of care. The RN becomes responsible, as the **manager of care**, to plan, implement, and evaluate the plan of care. This chapter assists you in gaining the tools necessary to be a strong manager of care within complex acute and extended-care settings.

Theoretical Framework

In the previous chapter you learned that Orem (2001) believes that individuals have self-care and dependent-care abilities (or agencies), which work together to meet regulatory functioning and developmental needs. At various times in life, a person will have a health care demand, either a self-care or dependent-care demand, which exceeds his or her **self-care agency**. When this happens, the person is said to have a self-care or dependent-care deficit. When this deficit is such that the person needs the specialized training of health care professionals, the person enters the health care setting and engages in a collaborative relationship with the RN and other health care team members.

Nurses have had specialized training to recognize the physiological, spiritual, social, emotional, and intellectual responses to illness states. Additionally, we understand that every medical, surgical, or nursing intervention has a **consequence**, which may be regarded as an outcome or a side effect. A consequence is any significant response to or effect of an intervention. An *outcome* is an expected consequence of an intervention and can be measured. An unexpected consequence is considered a *side effect* or adverse effect of an intervention.

Orem (2001) believes that the overall goal of nursing is to reestablish the health care agencies of the patient. The role of the acute care nurse has ended when the balance shifts away from the acute, dependent-care needs of the patient. The **dependent-care agency** returns to the patient or can be met by someone with other specific training to meet his or her short-term or extended needs beyond the acute care setting. The health care requirements within the **secondary (acute) health care** system are as follows (Orem, 2001, p. 131):

> (1) Prevention of complicating disease and adverse effects of specific disease and prolonged disability through early diagnosis and treatment (secondary treatment) and (2) rehabilitation in the event of disfigurement and disability (tertiary level of prevention) are specified in relation to what is known about the nature and effects of specific diseases, valid methods of regulating disease, and the human potential for living with and overcoming the disabling effects of disease.

Acute health care requirements vary with the progress of the disease either toward a cure or through complications that can occur. The RN uses information from many different sources to identify potential and actual problems with the patient's progress. The overall focus is to prevent complications while promoting a higher level of health (FYI 16-1). Figure 16-1 depicts the wealth of resources and abilities one has during health and the diminished nature of the same at the point where secondary and tertiary interventions are required.

The priority of care is unique and dynamic, or constantly changing, for each patient in the acute care setting. Patients are entering and leaving the acute care setting more dependent than in years past. The hospital setting is reserved for only the most acutely ill patients. Nurses are being increasingly challenged to understand and restore the individual self-care abilities for each individual. The primary role of the RN is to recognize

FYI 16-1 Secondary Care Outcome Priorities

The outcome priorities for a patient entering the acute (secondary) health care setting are as follows:

- Ensuring more independence in self-care ability
- Avoiding complications as the patient progresses through the illness state

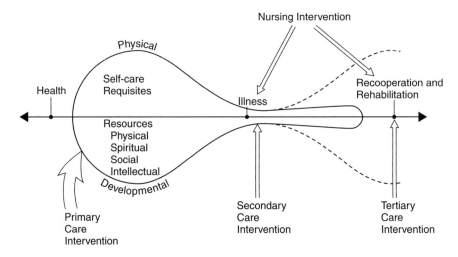

Figure 16-1 Primary, secondary, and tertiary care model.

when the patient's needs change, either to a more independent or dependent state. To best meet the needs of the patient and still use health care resources efficiently, the RN must continually reevaluate each patient against outcome criteria and determine the extent of the patient's dependent-care needs. When the priority of care warrants, the RN should advocate for a change in the level of health care.

Manager of Care

The RN manages the nursing and collaborative plan of care for the patient. The LPN works as a team member to carry out tasks, including assessment of the patient's response to the illness and the medical plan of care. These responses are communicated to the RN, who is then responsible for planning and modifying care to best meet the patient's needs. Since registered nurses are required to understand the pathophysiology and effects of disease, you will recognize such changes in the patient's condition as well as changes resulting from medication and other therapies used to treat the disease. You will manage the minute-to-minute and day-to-day changes that occur within multiple realms.

The manager of care must deal with unique problems that the acute care setting brings. These problems are associated with the technical and

> # FYI 16-2   Factors Influencing Patient Outcomes
>
> • Environment, both internal and external
> • Spiritual values and beliefs
> • Cultural values and beliefs
> • Developmental processes
> • Social roles and supports

institutional influences on the patient as well as the issues associated with the individual's environmental, spiritual, cultural, developmental, and social needs and influences (FYI 16-2).

Environmental Influences

Prior experience with the acute health care setting may affect a given patient in either a positive or a negative way. A patient who is familiar with the hospital routine and with a need for the equipment may respond better than the patient unfamiliar with the experience. Negative previous experiences, however, can make the patient more anxious. The RN must include interventions to orient the patient to the physical environment of the acute care setting and implement continuous assessment of the patient's response to the environment.

Much within the environment of the acute care setting has the potential to extend the patient's length of stay by introducing unexpected complications. Moving the patient through the acute care setting effectively and safely requires the RN to pay attention as the patient responds to the environment as well as to anticipate the potential effects the environment, including staffing issues, may have. A common nursing diagnosis is "potential for infection," and nosocomial, or hospital-acquired, infections are just one of the problems that competent nursing management can prevent. The charge nurse can manage this environmental concern by basing bed assignments on the diagnoses of the patients and then subsequently basing caregiver assignment on qualifications. For a patient likely to require more advanced intervention, the RN or LPN with the most experience will be assigned, whenever possible. However, newer nurses may be assigned more challenging patients when a more experienced nurse is available to assist.

Read the scenario in Exercise 16-1 and answer the questions concerning the environmental influences on a patient.

Spiritual Needs and Influences

Patients facing stressful health-care–related events may also experience **spiritual distress**. Illness states can place a patient in a position that

---

Exercise 16-1

A patient is admitted to an intensive care unit with a peripheral and central line, with a chest tube, and on a five-lead cardiac monitor. The family is asking about the alarms that are sounding from the monitor and from the IV pumps. The patient is quiet but appears anxious.

1. What questions would you ask to assess the environmental influence on the patient's recovery?

2. What outcomes would you have for this nursing diagnosis: "Coping, ineffective individual and family related to inexperience/knowledge deficit of the intensive care environment, as evidenced by anxious look, frequent questions regarding equipment and alarms"?

forces consideration of the fragile nature of life. Resulting from a potential life or death experience or a life-changing event, such as becoming paralyzed; losing a limb, sight, or hearing; or learning to live with a debilitating illness, spiritual distress may take on many manifestations. Much as in the grief process, the patient may display anger, blame, bargaining, or denial, or may overtly cling to a spiritual guide. As RN, you assess for spiritual distress and implement interventions that will help the patient cope, such as facilitating the patient's spiritual connection either through a referral or just by respecting personal wishes. Often the patient will require a spiritual guide by his or her side.

Additionally, religious beliefs may affect the patient's willingness to participate in the medical plan of care. For example, some religions forbid their participants from receiving blood or blood products. The plan of care must be respectful of the patient's beliefs while still providing the optimal environment for recovery.

According to Gorin and Arnold (1998), the effect spirituality has on health and well-being has not been studied extensively. An apparent link exists between the individual's ability to cope with adverse situations and his or her spiritual strength. Gorin and Arnold note that spirituality can even become stronger in times of adversity. In the acute care setting, we can easily overlook a person's spiritual needs when physical needs are evident. Be certain to attend to your patients in a holistic manner.

Cultural Needs and Influences

Culture affects how people respond to situations as a result of patterns acquired over time through social and religious structures as well as through their intellect and artistic expression (Giger & Davidhizar, 1995). Members of cultural groups typically share values, beliefs, norms, and practices. The acute care setting may place an individual in a position that involves conflict with beliefs. This **cultural strain** is the tension or pressure experienced by someone who has beliefs tested or when the actions of others are contrary to the beliefs, placing him or her in a position that potentially compromises these beliefs.

Cultural strain may be manifested in the patient's responses to the surroundings or to the plan of care. One culture-derived concept is personal space, the distance surrounding a person considered to be part of his or her identity. Personal space is generally thought to be between 1 and

3 feet around a person, depending on the cultural upbringing and personal interpretation. A breach of that space by objects or another person may cause discomfort and stress.

Within the acute care setting, the patient's personal space is often breached by the RN and other health care workers. Direct touching required during physical examinations may be the first experience the patient has with giving up personal space. Recognizing that the patient may have this concern requires the nurse to be respectful and seek permission to "invade the personal space," with adequate explanation of the need.

Respecting the patient's personal space also occurs during the interview stage. Some cultures require eye contact, but others may be offended by what they consider to be the presumptive nature of eye contact. Body language sometimes reveals patient discomfort with the interview process. Paying attention to the patient's comfort level during history taking will encourage the establishment of trust.

One patient may have grown up with family members with extensive hospitalization or illness, whereas another may have had minimal or no experience with the health care system. Additionally, since ideas about health and other values, including responses to the illness state, are largely formed within a particular culture, one patient may hide his or her emotions and another may wear emotions on his or her sleeve. However, they may equally be in despair. Cultural beliefs and subsequent behavior must be respected by the health care team to optimize a positive environment for healing. The RN who fails to respond to patients with equal respect can create mistrust of the plan of care as well as of the health care system.

Developmental Needs and Influences

While moving through life, everyone experiences developmental milestones. An acute or chronic illness state may pose a threat to the patient's developmental tasks. Many factors, such as stress from the illness state, uncertainty over long-term effects on self-care abilities, and perception of the plan of care, can pose a threat to the developmental tasks of the patient. "Role strain" is an appropriate nursing diagnosis when exploring a patient's concern over future or current developmental weaknesses. Outcome criteria focus on the return of the patient to as high a level of function as possible.

Social Needs and Influences

Humans, for the most part, are social beings. The acute care facility is a stressor to both patient and family. It can isolate the patient from the **social support** systems that he or she has in place. The needs of the family may not appear to be a priority for the nurse in planning the patient's care, but they must be considered for the patient to receive ample social support. The rest of the family is facing some of the same stresses as the hospitalized family member. They may need assistance coping with hospitalization of the patient or with the prospect of a poor prognosis (Appleyard et al, 2000; De Jong and Beatty, 2000; Gavaghan and Carroll, 2002; Kosco and Warren, 2000; Mendonca and Warren 1998; Tin, French, and Leung, 1999).

The family of a patient facing acute illness needs open, honest information about their hospitalized family member. The nurse should anticipate providing updates and other information without the family's having to solicit it, easing some of their concerns.

Family members need to be with the patient as much as possible. Allowing access, especially at times when the patient's prognosis may be poor, is an essential component to the plan of care. It will help both the family and the patient cope.

Monitoring the patient's response to family visitations is an important consideration for the RN. Often the family visits can be stressful to the patient rather than a source of comfort. Ensure that the patient's needs are held as the top priority. You may need to restrict visits on behalf of the patient.

Social support for the patient may come from others who are not legal relatives. Since people live and work within a community, friendships and companionship outside of family may become as important to someone as family. Many nontraditional definitions of family exist, which may include many combinations of significant individuals. Such nontraditional family relationships may present legal and ethical consequences within the acute care setting. For example, questions of confidentiality and privacy may need to be answered before planning care that includes keeping such people informed about the patient's progress.

The RN must recognize strain within the patient's social support system. "Ineffective individual or family coping, high risk for, related to multiple stress situations of hospitalization" would be a potential nursing diagnosis for patients experiencing decreased or ineffectual social support.

Resource Manager

As a manager of care within the acute care setting, you will be responsible for recognizing that limited funds are available to provide acute health care. Within the limits set by administration, staffing mixes, and restrictions on equipment and supplies, the RN must provide the patient with consistently safe and effective care, including managing resources. Each day a patient is in the hospital, valuable human, equipment, and supply resources are being used. The RN must then continue to evaluate the priority of care for each patient to advocate safe and efficient transitions to a less acute level of care.

Clinical Pathways

A **clinical pathway** is a standardized care map that defines nursing care, outcome criteria, and evaluation time frames for specific disorders. Clinical pathways are designed to manage the resources of the health care agency as well as enable consistent, safe care for patients. A clinical pathway defines the standard assessment data and frequency of the collection of the data needed for a specific illness or surgical procedure. These data include medical diagnostic tests, laboratory results, and vital signs, as well as fluid intake and output, for example. The pathway time frame also includes assessment points with defined outcome criteria. The responsibility of the RN is to evaluate the effectiveness of the plan of care and the patient's progress toward discharge.

Managing patient care requires the RN to ensure that the standard laboratory results, interventions, medications, and assessment data flow as outlined in the pathway. An RN learns to recognize and understand deviations from normal and is in a position, through collaboration with the physician and other health care team members, to adjust the plan of care to fit the individual needs of the patient. Strict adherence to evaluation points and efficient adjustments to the plan of care through collaboration will minimize the possibility of large deviations from the clinical pathway, which would increase the cost of care.

Discharge Planning

Patients moving through the acute care setting will eventually be discharged. The medical plan of care will have progressed to a point that the level of nursing care will have changed. The nursing plan of care will also change to a point that will require the RN to plan for discharge. In some facilities, discharge planning is a collaboration with the health care team and generally begins soon after admission. Patient outcome criteria are defined by the physician as well as the RN and are the source of evaluation of the patient's progress. If clinical pathways are used, then discharge dates may be identified as well.

Discharge planning requires assessing the patient plan of care to determine whether the outcome criteria are met. If a need exists for continuation of the plan of care, then the RN must evaluate whether the patient and family can continue with the necessary interventions or whether they need assistance. If the patient and the family are able to continue the plan of care, discharge teaching with regard to the continued care is needed. Discharge teaching will require the RN to assess the level of the patient's understanding with regard to his or her illness state and treatment regimen.

After discharge from an acute care facility, the patient may still need some level of nursing care or other specialized care beyond the patient's self-care ability, despite his or her having regained some independence. The physician will provide discharge orders that include the level of care needed. Occupational and physical therapy are continued for many patients discharged from acute care settings. Evaluation may reveal that a patient needs extended care.

Tertiary Care Referrals

The purposes of **tertiary care** are to provide health restoration and maintenance and to continue with health promotion (FYI 16-3). Health promotion and restoration assist the patient in achieving a higher level of functioning. For the patient with a progressive or terminal disorder, health maintenance focuses on at least sustaining the current level of functioning, slowing or preventing the effects of the disease. The goal of health maintenance is the establishment or continuation of dignity and respect during a condition of infirmity. By recognizing that the patient will require some level of dependent care, much effort must be taken to help the patient retain as much control and independence as possible. Review Figure 16-1 to note how tertiary interventions continue to expand the patient's resources and abilities for self-care.

FYI 16-3   **Tertiary Health Care**

- Tertiary health care involves health promotion and health maintenance.
- The outcome priority of tertiary health care is to ensure that the patient regains or attains as much independence as possible.

A patient to be discharged to an extended-care facility is generally evaluated by a caseworker, who is usually a social worker or an RN with special training to evaluate the needs and the extent of care requirements of the patient. The discharge RN notifies the caseworker and reports the patient's history of the present acute illness state along with the progress to date. The caseworker, having knowledge of the services within different facilities, makes recommendations and assists in making arrangements for transfer to the facility chosen. The caseworker considers the economic needs of the patient and assists families in managing insurance or other forms of payment for care.

The RN may need to make a referral to hospice care when a patient has approximately 6 months or less to live. Hospice care helps the patient and family cope with the end-of-life experience. The priority of care is the patient's peaceful and dignified death after living life, even its very end, to the fullest. The hospice nurse assesses the continued needs of the patient and works with a physician to provide comfort measures for the patients. Pain and nutrition are important components in managing a patient at the end of life.

A patient who leaves the hospital with a chronic illness state will perhaps go home under the care of the family. Chronic care of a patient can take a toll on other family members. Respite care, services provided by persons trained in the care of people with special needs, can be given within the home or through adult day care centers. It is intended to offer the patient's family members time off from their dependent-care duties.

Home health care provides assistance to a patient and family for a short period of time after discharge to home from the acute care setting. Home health care agencies provide a variety of care, depending on patient needs, such as physical therapy, respiratory therapy, or occupational therapy. Home health care is capable of providing health promotion, health restoration, and health maintenance care. The needs of the patient are generally assessed with an intake interview and assessment by an RN case manager. The level of care and the treatment plan are then determined accordingly.

Summary

Secondary, or acute, health care uses the principles of health restoration and health maintenance. A person seeks secondary care when in need of specialized, around-the-clock nursing care, having an imbalance between health care abilities and dependent-care needs. The RN is trained to take care of the patient's holistic needs on a minute-to-minute basis.

Continued-care needs of the patient are met within the varied realm of the tertiary health care system. In many cases, tertiary care is carried out either in long-term facilities or in the home with the assistance of both family and health care personnel. Both secondary and tertiary care needs are considered upon admission to a health care setting.

Critical Thinking Questions

1. A 74-year-old patient is admitted to an intensive care bed with a medical diagnosis of exacerbation of congestive heart failure and pulmonary edema. The patient has the following assessment data available: pulse 120-130 beats/min (A-Fib); respiration 26 breaths/min, labored, with crackles to the bases and coarse rhonchi throughout; oxygen per nasal cannula at 4 L, pulse oximetry 96%; 2+ pitting dependent edema bilateral lower extremities and to the coccyx area.

a. What further questions need to be asked?

b. What is the definitive care priority?

c. What patient problems are identified, and what are the outcome criteria?

d. Identify the developmental stage of the patient and the possible influence the disease response will have on the patient's perception of the future.

2. You enter your patient's room to do a shift assessment. The patient's family is gathered around the bed being led in prayer by a *curandera* (faith healer). The room is decorated with candles and religious paraphernalia. The ritual has a supernatural feel, and the patient is being offered a potent herbal tea mix.

a. What questions do you need to ask?

    b. What interventions, if any, are necessary?

    c. To what extent would you report or chart the findings?

3. A patient is to receive an IVPB of 20 mEq K+ in a bolus for a K+ level of 3.0. On hand you have an IVPB of 20 mEq in 100 ml of 0.9% NS. The K+ should be run no faster than 10 mEq/hr.

    a. At what setting would you place the pump to comply with the recommended IV rate?

    b. The patient complains that the IV is burning, and on assessment the IV site is red and slightly raised. What is your next step?

    c. The lab has been notified to draw a K+ level 1 hour after the finish of the IVPB. You have already put in the order for the lab to draw 3 hours after the initial start. What action would be correct at this point?

References

Appleyard ME et al: Nurse-coached interventions for the families of patients in critical care units, *Crit Care Nurse* 20(3):40, 2000.

De Jong MJ, Beatty DS: Family perceptions of support interventions in the intensive care unit, *Dimens Crit Care Nurs* 19(5):40, 2000.

Gavaghan SR, Carroll DL: Families of critically ill patients and the effects of nursing intervention, *Dimens Crit Care Nurs* 21(2):64, 2002.

Giger JN, Davidhizar RE: *Transcultural nursing: assessment and intervention*, ed 2, St Louis, 1995, Mosby.

Gorin SS, Arnold J: *Health promotion handbook*, St Louis, 1998, Mosby.

Kosco M, Warren NA: Critical care nurses' perceptions of family needs as met, *Crit Care Nurs Q* 23(2):60, 2000.

Mendonca D, Warren N: Perceived and unmet needs of critical care family members, *Crit Care Nurs Q* 21(1):58, 1998.

Orem DE: *Nursing concepts of practice*, ed 6, St Louis, 2001, Mosby.

Tin MK, French P, Leung KK: The needs of the family of critically ill neurosurgical patients: a comparison of nurses' and family members' perceptions, *J Neurosci Nurs* 31(6):348, 1999.

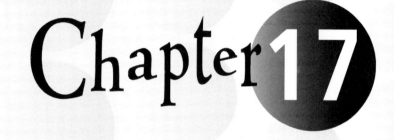

Chapter 17

Putting It All Together

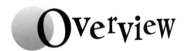Overview

Change takes effort. You have decided to make a major change in your life and have put forth effort to get to where you are in the process of becoming an RN. Along the way you have been given tools necessary to make the change. You have been asked to set forth a plan to assist you through your program of study.

This chapter uses the nursing process to assist you in reflecting on your journey thus far and to challenge you to develop a portfolio, a map to your future. You will reassess your strengths and weaknesses, make a diagnosis, plan goals, decide what tools you will need to implement your plan, identify what might be stopping you from progressing or ways you are enduring, and evaluate your readiness to embark upon the next leg of your journey. If you set a course for excellence and have a lamp to light your way, then the road to success will not seem so difficult to travel.

Assessment

In Chapter 1 you were asked to "sketch your experiential resume." You were asked to look at this resume and determine experiences with positive and negative influences on your learning. After defining yourself, you identified and prioritized short-term and long-term personal and professional goals and your personal-care priority. You finalized your plan with a timeline for meeting these goals.

In the journey you have taken to this point, you have had the opportunity to learn and use new tools and expand your horizon through a broader base of knowledge. Brown and Gillis (1999) report that reflective thinking is an effective method for students to develop professional and personal philosophies. Development of a professional philosophy is an important component for the transition of a student with no nursing background into the role of professional nurse. The LPN mobility student, also being in a role transition, would benefit from reflective thinking to develop a personal and professional philosophy as well. Brown and Gillis demonstrate the relationship between reflective thinking and critical thinking. Through their literature search, the authors show how reflection is a dynamic process of analysis that forces the student to examine prejudices, beliefs, feelings, thoughts, and experiences in light of new nursing knowledge. Consider the process of reflection as a proactive way to challenge former assumptions and inferences about the role of the RN.

Critical Reflection

To begin critical reflection, you must ask yourself tough questions about your beliefs. What are the differences between your beliefs about the role of the RN from what you know of the role of the LPN? If you answer truthfully, you will be able to identify areas for needed role development. Del Bueno (2000) remarks that the beginning RN must meet a minimum set of competencies to be safe in the new role:

1. Ability to recognize problems from presenting signs and symptoms
2. Awareness of the urgency of a situation and acting appropriately to the level of urgency
3. Capacity to design a plan of care that safely meets the needs of the patient
4. Understanding the nature of the plan of care in relationship to the patient's medical and nursing problems

Additional competencies of the beginning RN include strong interpersonal skills (teamwork, team building, conflict resolution, and patient interactions) and a competent level of clinical skills (del Bueno, 2000). The implications to you as a soon-to-be graduate are out in the "real world," without the safety net of school. You will be asked to apply the knowledge, skills, and values you have learned in order to be a safe and effective practitioner.

Within the academic setting, you will demonstrate sufficient knowledge and skill to manage several patients in a safe, holistic manner. The graduate RN leaves school with the knowledge and skills of a generalist within the nursing profession. However, the journey of learning and skill acquisition is far from over. Your professional development begins with a reflection on your past as a means to better understand the lessons you have learned. The philosophy of nursing you develop will serve as the basis for your future plan. Use Exercise 17-1 to begin the reflective process.

When you began your journey to becoming an RN, you may have wanted to know more about the nursing care you were giving, what the signs and symptoms meant, and how the plan of care would affect your

Exercise 17-1

A patient presents to you with the following signs and symptoms: blood pressure 148/60 mm Hg, pulse 140 beats/min, respirations 18 breaths/min and deep with a fruity odor, blood sugar 485; lethargic, with slurring speech; and flushed and warm.

Ask yourself these questions: Are you able to recognize patient problems from the presenting signs and symptoms? Do you understand the significance and urgency of the patient information? Can you design a plan of care that effectively manages the patient problems and will assist the patient toward health? Do you know the reasons behind your nursing plan and the medical plan of care, and the relationship between the presenting patient signs and symptoms and problems?

When you are done with this brief evaluation, form a group in class where you can discuss your findings and defend yourself.

What assumptions that you made were not supported by the data presented?

Did you make any prejudicial assumptions?

How did these assumptions influence your plan of care?

patients' outcomes. This curiosity is as important now as it was then. Curiosity will lead you to continued education, which will improve your nursing care. Understanding the relationship of the disease process to the interventions provided by nursing and by other members of the health care team will help you become a safe practitioner. The standard of practice for all nurses is to become an informed caregiver who is able to recognize significant changes in patient conditions, anticipate needs, and implement appropriate interventions.

In Exercise 17-2 and after reviewing the plan you developed in Chapter 1, begin a retrospective assessment of where you are to date. You may be near graduation, or you may be further off yet one semester closer to graduation. Either way, hopefully your course of study and this textbook have provided you with new insights.

From the problems you identified in Exercise 17-2, which ones are priorities to you? Did you choose improvements that will enhance your critical thinking abilities, broaden your knowledge base, and help with your skills? You need to recognize areas that pertain to your most immediate needs first, as well as ensure your ability to provide safe care. Remember that critical reflection is unbiased and does not let your ego interfere with the search for truth.

In planning care, pointing out and leveraging strengths is as important as identifying and correcting weaknesses. Capitalize on your strengths in your plan of action as tools to be built upon. In Exercise 17-3, read the scenario and answer the questions about your strengths and weaknesses.

Your strengths will also assist you in your quest to become the best you can be. Clustering the strengths across from the weaknesses (see Exercise 17-2), can you identify how you will be able to draw from them to assist you in gaining experience and expertise? As an LPN, many treatment skills have become second nature to you. As a graduate from a mobility program, not needing to concentrate on practicing basic psychomotor skills, you will be more open to the evolving changes in the conditions that define the needs of your patient. Thus your unique set of strengths has enhanced a critical component of your ability to provide safe, effective care.

Making the Diagnosis

In clustering your strengths and weaknesses (see Exercise 17-2), you have a chance to identify diagnostic statements. These problem (or strength)

Exercise 17-2

Strengths (Gifts)	Weaknesses (Barriers)

How have your strengths and weaknesses changed since you listed them in Chapter 2?

Write a problem statement for each of your weaknesses:

Weakness	Problem Statement

Which of these problems are priorities for you to resolve?

areas will assist you in continued planning. If you have kept a journal, review it to see whether the problem areas that you have identified in Exercise 17-2 are part of your past problem list. If so, a revision of a pre-existing plan of action may be all that is needed. A self-diagnosis should be specific to the problem, as should a plan to capitalize on and extend a strength. For example, if you have determined that you are not sure of all of the signs and symptoms to expect from a patient experiencing an exacerbation of a disorder, then your problem statement might be written like this: "Cognitive deficit, inability to identify pertinent data to make sound

Exercise 17-3

Hypothetically, consider that you have difficulty finding the correct way to interact with a patient or family member who is having trouble coping with hospitalization or illness. You may decide that this reflects a problem with your own ability to effectively use the catchphrases that are a part of therapeutic communication. You feel that your strength lies in recognizing that people need to have someone to talk with who is empathetic, but you feel awkward trying to be that someone.

1. How would you state the problems, and what would they be related to?

2. How would you go about using the strength you identified to assist you with weaknesses you've identified?

3. Is there a catchphrase that you can believe in that will allow you to display empathy?

4. Is there a way for you to show empathy while also calling on another health care team member, such as the chaplain, to assist the patient in this time of need?

Continued

5. What steps would you take to improve your communication skills?

clinical judgment." As in any diagnostic statement, you should identify what the problem is related to. A problem can be resolved only after you know the reasons behind it.

What could the problem's cause be for you? You might have worked too much at your job and not had enough time to study. You may have chosen to settle for a minimum grade point average or study for a specific test, rather than seeking deep understanding and true knowledge. Whatever the cause of the problem, you should be honest in conducting your critical reflection. Determining a problem's cause, or at least conditions that seem to lead to the problem, should assist you in developing a plan that focuses on your problem areas.

In Exercise 17-2, you created problem statements that apply to those areas of weakness. Prioritize the problems to develop a plan to work on the problems of greatest importance first. You may need to solicit the advice of a faculty member or your mentor in making decisions on how to prioritize.

Planning

Now is the time to formulate personal and professional goals that will assist you with the transition into your new role as a safe beginning RN. Use the weaknesses you identified in Exercise 17-2 as problem areas to establish goals and outcome criteria. As in Chapter 1, establish your short-term and long-term goals. Short-term goals may assist you in meeting the needs of your family, seeking a job, or getting oriented to a new town, as well as passing the NCLX-RN exam. Long-term goals can assist you during the orientation period in establishing and maintaining your mentor relationship and planning your future education. Long-term goals will also assist you in your professional development, such as planning for certification in a specialty area, earning an advanced degree—even becoming an advanced practice nurse (APN). The destination is yours to determine.

Professional development is an expected part of the role of the RN, yet being a professional is more than being licensed as an RN. Becoming a professional means establishing yourself as capable, competent, and safe. It also means that you act to advance the practice of nursing through your actions and your skills. Orem (2001) defines *profession* in nursing as "the basis for distinguishing nurses prepared for entry to the beginning professional level of nursing practice who move themselves to become advanced professional practitioners from nurses prepared in technical programs preparatory for nursing" (p. 465). The LPN is trained at the technical level, and the RN receives education at the beginning professional level. Orem's definition implies that your professional development includes an obligation to advance yourself within the practice of nursing and does not stop at the end of your formal educational process. To be a part of the profession of nursing, you must set goals that advance your professional development, building up your knowledge, skill, and critical thinking abilities.

In Exercise 17-4, write your personal and professional goals and outcome criteria associated with the goals. Include a personal development plan that is in balance with your professional plan. You should reestablish personal relationships to help cope with the transition into your new role. You might have neglected those closest to you during your schooling. The stress and pressure to complete a program that is abbreviated may have left you little time to spend with family and friends. Once-important relaxation activities, such as exercise, hobbies, and entertainment, might have been set aside while you were concentrating on your RN education. Remember, your self-definition is more than as an RN, for you may be a mother or father, sister or brother, potter, sewer, triathlete, actor, and friend. All the aspects of who you are help make you a better RN.

Implementation

Now that you have set your goals, you can implement your plan of action. Interventions to achieve your goals will assist you in establishing discipline and dedication to your professional development. Reflect on the interventions that assisted you in achieving your goal to graduate from your nursing

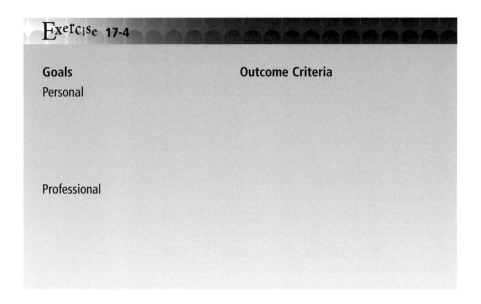

Exercise 17-4

Goals	Outcome Criteria
Personal	
Professional	

program. Add to those interventions that assisted you in achieving your goal new interventions derived from the tools you have learned.

Remember to set time aside each day as study time. As a new graduate, your studying will be focused on the common patient problems presented in your work environment. You should also focus on reviewing for the NCLEX-RN exam. Will you take a review course or buy review books? Both? Will you form a study circle, or are you a solitary learner?

Your interventions will be unique for you. However, certain common interventions can be helpful in your role transition. Since learning is better when it has direct application or when it will be used soon after it has taken place, one intervention is to request a patient assignment that complements your area of need. You will learn more about complications of hypertension, for example, if you take a patient with hypertension than if you just read about them. Another way to enhance your knowledge base is to ask your mentor or preceptor questions that help you understand how he or she arrived at a conclusion or decision.

Your New Tools

In approaching graduation, you bring with you many new tools related to knowledge, skills, and values. List these tools in Exercise 17-5. Cluster

Exercise 17-5

Tool	Maintenance Plan

these tools into categories, such as those you may use daily, weekly, or occasionally. If you find a tool or skill that you might use infrequently, how will you maintain expertise with it? Competency requires that you maintain currency in all aspects of your job. All aspects of the RN's role must be carried out safely and with the utmost proficiency. To ensure patient satisfaction and positive outcomes, if you are called upon to start an intravenous line, for example, your proficiency will decrease patient stress and minimize risks.

What's Stopping You?

You have demonstrated commitment in your journey through the educational process. You have learned much along the way and are now ready to begin your new role, but are you truly ready to take on your new role? Have you subconsciously or even consciously set up barriers that keep you from moving into your new role?

Change can provoke anxiety, especially at the initiation of a whole new direction in life. Within your nursing program, you have been guided and had a safety net. Now you are going to be making decisions on your own, with patients and a team depending on you. You will be required to manage care based on the soundness of your knowledge and skills. This alone could be a source of anxiety and could give you pause. Yet keep in mind the "gifts" you have gained, the knowledge and the tools you have. This will assist you in gaining confidence.

In Exercise 17-6, list the barriers you have identified that may be keeping you from doing your best. Next to each, state what you can do to break through the barrier.

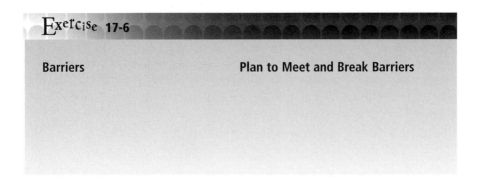

Barriers	Plan to Meet and Break Barriers

Confidence will come with experience. You must overcome the urge to resist change and continue in the more comfortable role of the LPN. An RN who is not accepting the need to change is placing patients at risk. You have learned that the RN is an advocate for patients and as an advocate must know how to make decisions that are sound and safe.

In your role as an LPN, you have had to rely on the RN to make patient care decisions. You may have known an RN who made poor decisions and many more who made correct decisions. As an LPN, you may even have believed that you could have solved a problem better than the RN. Now you have the power and the responsibility to make these decisions. What image do you want to project to the LPN who will be working with you?

Evaluation

Until now you have assessed your readiness, what you have learned, and how your philosophy has changed. Now it is up to you to evaluate the effectiveness of your efforts to become an RN. You have many ways in which to evaluate yourself. You can take an emotional inventory, asking during your orientation period whether you are ready to accept the emotional roller-coaster ride associated with the RN role. You may need to do a confidence inventory as well. How confident are you? You have acquired the tools necessary; now it is up to you to say, "I can do the job." Confidence will come with experience and with an established support system, such as a mentor, your family, or another significant person. Take a moment to complete Exercise 17-7, a tool that will help you make the transition to the RN role.

NCLEX-RN Preparation

Many review courses, computer programs, and books are designed to evaluate your readiness for the NCLEX-RN exam. Your college will likely require a specific exam that you and your classmates will take. You may be able to borrow many other tests from the library or purchase them on the Internet. In any case, this is a critical step in preparing for the NCLEX-RN exam.

As you think back about your years in nursing school, what subject areas did you find the most difficult, perhaps psychiatric nursing or maternal-child health nursing? Was pharmacology a mystery to you, or math? Do you still sometimes struggle with dosage calculations or remembering which classification of drugs does what? Don't panic. Evaluate where you need improvement and create a plan of action, just as you would for your patients.

Each of your strengths and weaknesses defines where you are in your educational process. As an RN, you are expected to be a generalist, able to care for a patient presenting with several different problems and with several different responses to treatment. Therefore pay attention to the areas on your NCLEX-RN readiness exam that bring back those not-so-great memories of difficult learning experiences. Then set your sights on doing something about your deficit. You can do it!

Exercise 17-7

On a piece of paper—heavy, colored construction paper if you choose—trace your right or left hand, and then cut around the tracing. Now decorate the cutout hand, using encouraging words or phrases or bright and cheerful pictures. When you are satisfied with your creation, take the hand and mount it on the jamb of a door through which you will go at the beginning of every day and at the end of the day. Each time you pass the hand, give yourself a pat on the back and say to yourself, "I did a good job today" or "I am doing a good job and deserve to tell myself so." No matter how tough the day will get, you should commend yourself and recognize the positive parts of your day. For each of the self-improvements you plan to make, find at least one strength or strategy that will get you there.

Summary

This chapter was intended to help you evaluate your journey through the transition from LPN to RN. You were asked to reflect on your journey as a means to identify your philosophy of nursing as an RN. Take the philosophy you have developed in writing and tuck away the paper in a safe place. When you have doubts about what you are doing or why you are doing it, take the paper out and read it. See whether your philosophy has changed or whether you have forgotten some of the tools you had learned. As you journey through the rest of your RN career, your philosophy of nursing will likely evolve. Embrace the possibilities that a career in nursing, a life of nursing, has to offer, and do what you are called to do.

Critical Thinking Questions

Now you can develop your own critical thinking questions. Begin with a case scenario from your clinical experience. Consider the signs and symptoms and disease process. What assessments do you need to make? Review Chapter 9 to assist you with determining what questions to ask. Develop a plan of care and make a prediction as to when your patient should reach the intended outcomes. Evaluate the effectiveness of the plan and explain the reasons for the outcomes that actually occurred.

References

Brown SC, Gillis MA: Using reflective thinking to develop personal professional philosophies, *J Nurs Educ* 38(4):171, 1999.

del Bueno DJ: *A model for competence and success,* presentation at Northeast Baptist Hospital, San Antonio, Tex, March 2000.

Orem DE: *Nursing: concepts of practice,* ed 6, St Louis, 2001, Mosby.

Appendix A

Math Review
Post-Test

1. The physician orders digoxin 0.375 mg PO once daily. Digoxin is supplied in 0.25 mg tablets. How many tablets do you give?

2. The physician orders amoxicillin 0.5 g PO tid. The antibiotic is supplied in 250 mg capsules. How many capsules do you give per dose?

3. The physician orders levothyroxine 0.025 mg PO daily. The medication is supplied in 50 μg tablets. How many tablets do you give per dose?

4. The physician orders warfarin 7.5 mg PO daily at bedtime. The medication is supplied in 5 mg tablets. How many tablets do you give per dose?

5. The physician orders 20 mEq potassium chloride PO daily × 3. The medication is supplied in liquid form with a concentration of 10 mEq/5 ml. How many milliliters do you give per dose?

6. Your patient is experiencing chest pain, and the standing physician order for this patient in the event of chest pain is nitroglycerin 0.6 mg sublingually. The medication is supplied in 1/100 gr per tablet. How many tablets do you give?

7. The physician orders nystatin 250,000 U, swish and swallow, tid. The medication is supplied in an oral suspension of 100,000 U/ml. How many ml do you give?

8. The physician orders paroxetine 30 mg daily. The medication is supplied in scored 20 mg tablets. How many tablets do you give?

9. The physician orders celecoxib 200 mg PO daily. The medication is supplied in 100 mg capsules. How many capsules do you give?

10. The physician orders azithromycin suspension 200 mg on day 1 and 100 mg on days 2, 3, 4, and 5. The medication is supplied in a 15 ml bottle with a concentration of 200 mg/5 ml. How many tsp do you give on day 1? How many tsp do you give on subsequent days?

11. The physician orders heparin 5000 U SC. The medication is supplied in a concentration of 10,000 U/ml. How many ml do you give?

12. The physician orders morphine sulfate 30 mg IM q8h prn. The medication is supplied in a concentration of 15 mg/ml. How many ml do you give?

13. The physician orders phytonadione 5 mg SC × 1. The medication is supplied in a concentration of 10 mg/ml. How many ml do you give?

14. The physician orders meperidine 50 mg IM q4h prn. The medication is supplied in a concentration of 100 mg/ml. How many ml do you give?

15. The physician orders furosemide 30 mg slow IVP × 1. The medication is supplied in a concentration of 40 mg/4 ml. How many ml do you give?

16. The physician orders methylprednisolone 100 mg IM × 1. The medication is supplied in a concentration of 500 mg/ml. How many ml do you give?

17. The physician orders secobarbital 100 mg IM × 1 only 30 minutes before a procedure. The medication is supplied in a concentration of 50 mg/ml. How many ml do you give?

18. The physician orders erythropoietin 75 U/kg SC three times weekly. Your patient weighs 150 pounds. The medication is supplied in a concentration of 10,000 U/ml. How many ml do you give?

19. The physician orders cefazolin 1 g IV q8h to be infused over 30 minutes. The medication is supplied in a concentration of 1000 mg/50 ml. Assuming a drip factor of 10 gtt/ml, how many gtt/min should infuse?

20. The physician orders 1 L D$_5$W to infuse over 12 hours. The drip factor is 10 gtt/ml. How many gtt/min should infuse?

21. The physician orders 1 L NS to infuse at 60 ml/hr. The drip factor is 15 gtt/ml. How many gtt/min should infuse?

22. The physician orders D$_5$ 1/2 NS to infuse at 80 ml/hr. The drip factor is 20 gtt/min. How many gtt/min should infuse?

23. The physician orders 1 L D$_5$RL to infuse over 8 hours. The drip factor is 60 gtt/ml. How many gtt/min should infuse?

24. The physician orders 0.5 L NS to infuse over 2 hours. The drip factor is 15 gtt/ml. How many gtt/min should infuse?

25. The physician orders NS at KVO (15 ml/hr in this case). The drip factor is 10 gtt/ml. How many gtt/min should infuse?

26. The physician orders 1 L NS to infuse over 10 hours. After 4 hours you note that only 200 ml has infused. The drip factor is 15 gtt/ml. What was the original rate of infusion in gtt/min? What is the recalculated rate after 4 hours?

27. The physician orders 1 L D_5W to infuse over 8 hours. After 3 hours you note that only 150 ml has infused. The drip factor is 10 gtt/ml. What was the original rate of infusion in gtt/min? What is the recalculated rate after 3 hours?

28. The physician orders 0.5 L 1/2NS to infuse over 4 hours. After 1 hour you note that only 75 ml has infused. The drip factor is 20 gtt/ml. What was the original infusion rate in gtt/min? What is the recalculated infusion rate after 1 hour?

29. The physician orders 0.5 L D_5W to infuse at 40 ml/hr. If the IV was started at 10 AM, when will it be finished?

30. The physician orders 1 g metronidazole (Flagyl IV) to be infused over 1 hour. The medication is supplied 1000 mg/100 ml. The drip factor is 20gtt/ml. How many gtt/min should infuse?

Answers

1. 1.5 tablets
2. 2 capsules
3. 0.5 tablet
4. 1.5 tablets
5. 10 ml
6. 1 tablet
7. 2.5 ml
8. 1.5 tablets
9. 2 capsules
10. 5 ml, 2.5 ml
11. 0.5 ml
12. 2 ml
13. 0.5 ml
14. 0.5 ml
15. 3 ml
16. 0.2 ml
17. 2 ml
18. 0.51 ml
19. 17 gtt/min
20. 14 gtt/min
21. 15 gtt/min
22. 27 gtt/min
23. 125 gtt/min
24. 63 gtt/min
25. 2.5 gtt/min
26. 25 gtt/min, 33 gtt/min
27. 21 gtt/min, 28 gtt/min
28. 42 gtt/min, 47 gtt/min
29. 10:30 PM
30. 33 gtt/min

Appendix B

A Patient's Bill of Rights

Introduction

Effective health care requires collaboration between patients and physicians and other health care professionals. Open and honest communication, respect for personal and professional values, and sensitivity to differences are integral to optimal patient care. As the setting for the provision of health services, hospitals must provide a foundation for understanding and respecting the rights and responsibilities of patients, their families, physicians, and other caregivers. Hospitals must ensure a health care ethic that respects the role of patients in decision making about treatment choices and other aspects of their care. Hospitals must be sensitive to cultural, racial, linguistic, religious, age, gender, and other differences, as well as the needs of persons with disabilities.

The American Hospital Association presents A *Patient's Bill of Rights* with the expectation that it will contribute to more effective patient care and be supported by the hospital on behalf of the institution and its medical staff, employees, and patients. The American Hospital Association encourages health care institutions to tailor the bill of rights to their patient community by translating and/or simplifying the language of the bill of rights as may be necessary to ensure that patients and their families understand their rights and responsibilities.

Bill of Rights*

1. The patient has the right to considerate and respectful care.
2. The patient has the right to and is encouraged to obtain from physicians and other direct caregivers relevant, current, and understandable information concerning diagnosis, treatment, and prognosis.

    Except in emergencies when the patient lacks decision-making capacity and the need for treatment is urgent, the patient is entitled to the opportunity to discuss and request information related to the specific procedures and/or treatments, the risks involved, the possible

---

*These rights can be exercised on the patient's behalf by a designated surrogate or proxy decision maker if the patient lacks decision-making capacity, is legally incompetent, or is a minor.

Reprinted with permission of the American Hospital Association, Copyright 1992.

length of recuperation, and the medically reasonable alternatives and their accompanying risks and benefits.

Patients have the right to know the identity of physicians, nurses, and others involved in their care, as well as when those involved are students, residents, or other trainees. The patient also has the right to know the immediate and long-term financial implications of treatment choices, insofar as they are known.

3. The patient has the right to make decisions about the plan of care prior to and during the course of treatment and to refuse a recommended treatment of plan of care to the extent permitted by law and hospital policy and to be informed of the medical consequences of this action. In case of such refusal, the patient is entitled to other appropriate care and services that the hospital provides or transfer to another hospital. The hospital should notify patients of any policy that might affect patient choice within the institution.

4. The patient has the right to have an advance directive (such as living will, health care proxy, or durable power of attorney for health care) concerning treatment or designating a surrogate decision maker with the expectation that the hospital will honor the intent of that directive to the extent permitted by law and hospital policy.

Health care institutions must advise patients of their rights under state law and hospital policy to make informed medical choices, ask if the patient has an advance directive, and include that information in patient records. The patient has the right to timely information about hospital policy that may limit its ability to implement fully a legally valid advance directive.

5. The patient has the right to every consideration of privacy. Case discussion, consultation, examination, and treatment should be conducted so as to protect each patient's privacy.

6. The patient has the right to expect that all communications and records pertaining to his or her care will be treated as confidential by the hospital, except in cases such as suspected abuse and public health hazards when reporting is permitted or required by law. The patient has the right to expect that the hospital will emphasize the confidentiality of this information when it releases it to any other parties entitled to review information in these records.

7. The patient has the right to review the records pertaining to his or her medication care and to have the information explained or interpreted as necessary, except when restricted by law.

8. The patient has the right to expect that, within its capacity and policies, a hospital will make reasonable response to the request of a patient for appropriate and medically indicated care and services. The hospital must provide evaluation, services, and/or referral as indicated by the urgency of the case. When medically appropriate and legally permissible, or when a patient has so requested, a patient may be transferred to another facility. The institution to which the patient is to be transferred must first have accepted the patient for transfer. The patient must also have the benefit of complete information and explanation concerning the need for risks, benefits, and alternatives to such a transfer.

9. The patient has the right to ask and be informed of the existence of business relationships among the hospital, educational institutions, other health care providers, or payers that may influence the patient's treatment and care.

10. The patient has the right to consent to or decline to participate in proposed research studies or human experimentation affecting care and treatment or requiring direct patient involvement, and to have those studies fully explained prior to consent. A patient who declines to participate in research or experimentation is entitled to the most effective care that the hospital can otherwise provide.

11. The patient has the right to expect reasonable continuity of care when appropriate and to be informed by physicians and other caregivers of available and realistic patient care options when hospital care is no longer appropriate.

12. The patient has the right to be informed of hospital policies and practices that relate to patient care, treatment, and responsibilities. The patient has the right to be informed of available resources for resolving disputes, grievances, and conflicts, such as ethics committees, patient representatives, or other mechanisms available in the institution. The patient has the right to be informed of the hospital's charges for services and available payment methods.

The collaborative nature of health care requires that patients, or their families or surrogates, participate in their care. The effectiveness of care and patient satisfaction with the course of treatment depend, in part, on the patient fulfilling certain responsibilities. Patients are responsible for providing information about past illnesses, hospitalizations, medications, and other matters related to health status. To participate effectively in decision making, patients must be encouraged to take responsibility for requesting additional information or clarification about their health status or treatment when they do not fully understand information and instructions. Patients are also responsible for informing their physicians and other caregivers if they anticipate problems in following prescribed treatment.

Patients should also be aware of the hospital's obligation to be reasonably efficient and equitable in providing care to other patients and the community. The hospital's rules and regulations are designed to help the hospital meet this obligation. Patients and their families are responsible for making reasonable accommodations to the needs of the hospital, other patients, medical staff, and hospital employees. Patients are responsible for providing necessary information for insurance claims and for working with the hospital to make payment arrangements, when necessary.

A person's health depends on much more than health care services. Patients are responsible for recognizing the influence of their lifestyle on their personal health.

Conclusion

Hospitals have many functions to perform, including the enhancement of health status, health promotion, and the prevention and treatment of injury and disease; the immediate and ongoing care and rehabilitation of patients; the education of health professionals, patients, and the community; and research. All these activities must be conducted with an overriding concern for the values and dignity of the patients.

Appendix C

NANDA Nursing Diagnoses 2001–2002

Activity intolerance
Activity intolerance, risk for
Adjustment, impaired
Airway clearance, ineffective
Allergy response, latex
Allergy response, risk for latex
Anxiety
Anxiety, death
Aspiration, risk for
Attachment, risk for impaired parent/infant/child
Autonomic dysreflexia
Autonomic dysreflexia, risk for
Body image, disturbed
Body temperature, risk for imbalanced
Bowel incontinence
Breastfeeding, effective
Breastfeeding, ineffective
Breastfeeding, interrupted
Breathing pattern, ineffective
Cardiac output, decreased
Caregiver role strain
Caregiver role strain, risk for
Communication, impaired verbal
Conflict, decisional
Conflict, parental role
Confusion, acute
Confusion, chronic
Constipation
Constipation, perceived
Constipation, risk for
Coping, ineffective
Coping, ineffective community
Coping, readiness for enhanced community
Coping, defensive
Coping, compromised family
Coping, disabled family
Coping, readiness for enhanced family
Denial, ineffective
Dentition, impaired

Development, risk for delayed
Diarrhea
Disuse syndrome, risk for
Diversional activity, deficient
Energy field, disturbed
Environmental interpretation syndrome, impaired
Failure to thrive, adult
Falls, risk for
Family processes, dysfunctional: alcoholism
Family processes, interrupted
Fatigue
Fear
Fluid volume, deficient
Fluid volume, excess
Fluid volume, risk for deficient
Fluid volume, risk for imbalanced
Gas exchange, impaired
Grieving, anticipatory
Grieving, dysfunctional
Growth and development, delayed
Growth, risk for disproportionate
Health maintenance, ineffective
Health-seeking behaviors
Home maintenance, impaired
Hopelessness
Hyperthermia
Hypothermia
Identity, disturbed personal
Incontinence, functional urinary
Incontinence, reflex urinary
Incontinence, stress urinary
Incontinence, total urinary
Incontinence, urge urinary
Incontinence, risk for urge urinary
Infant behavior, disorganized
Infant behavior, risk for disorganized
Infant behavior, readiness for enhanced organized
Infant feeding pattern, ineffective
Infection, risk for

Injury, risk for
Injury, risk for perioperative-positioning
Intracranial adaptive capacity, decreased
Knowledge, deficient
Loneliness, risk for
Memory, impaired
Mobility, impaired bed
Mobility, impaired physical
Mobility, impaired wheelchair
Nausea
Neglect, unilateral
Noncompliance
Nutrition, imbalanced: less than body requirements
Nutrition, imbalanced: more than body requirements
Nutrition, risk for imbalanced: more than body requirements
Oral mucous membrane, impaired
Pain, acute
Pain, chronic
Parenting, impaired
Parenting, risk for impaired
Peripheral neurovascular dysfunction, risk for
Poisoning, risk for
Post-trauma syndrome
Post-trauma syndrome, risk for
Powerlessness
Powerlessness, risk for
Protection, ineffective
Rape-trauma syndrome
Rape-trauma syndrome: compound reaction
Rape-trauma syndrome: silent reaction
Relocation stress syndrome
Relocation stress syndrome, risk for
Role performance, ineffective
Self-care deficit, bathing/hygiene
Self-care deficit, dressing/grooming
Self-care deficit, feeding
Self-care deficit, toileting
Self-esteem, chronic low
Self-esteem, situational low

Self-esteem, risk for situational low
Self-mutilation
Self-mutilation, risk for
Sensory perception, disturbed
Sexual dysfunction
Sexuality patterns, ineffective
Skin integrity, impaired
Skin integrity, risk for impaired
Sleep deprivation
Sleep pattern, disturbed
Social interaction, impaired
Social isolation
Sorrow, chronic
Spiritual distress
Spiritual distress, risk for
Spiritual well-being, readiness for enhanced
Suffocation, risk for
Suicide, risk for
Surgical recovery, delayed
Swallowing, impaired
Therapeutic regimen management, effective
Therapeutic regimen management, ineffective
Therapeutic regimen management, ineffective community
Therapeutic regimen management, ineffective family
Thermoregulation, ineffective
Thought processes, disturbed
Tissue integrity, impaired
Tissue perfusion, ineffective
Transfer ability, impaired
Trauma, risk for
Urinary elimination, impaired
Urinary retention
Ventilation, impaired spontaneous
Ventilatory weaning response, dysfunctional
Violence, risk for other-directed
Violence, risk for self-directed
Walking, impaired
Wandering

Index

Page numbers followed by f indicate figures; b, boxes.

as teacher, 215–233. *See also*
  Patient education;
  Teaching.
vs Licensed Practical Nurse
  (LPN), 106–109
Reliability, of research results, 264
Research, 256, 257
  communicating results in,
    265–266
  concepts in, 257–258
  data collection in, 263–264,
    265
  defining variables in, 259
  design of, 261–262
  hypothesis making in, 261
  importance of, 256
  interpreting results in, 265
  literature search in, 259, 261
  performance improvement, 257
  population definition in, 263
  quality assurance, 257
  reliability of, 264
  results of
    communicating, 265–266
    interpreting, 265
  sample selection in, 263
  topics for, 268
  using, in nursing process,
    256–257
  validity of, 264–265
  variables in, 258–259
Research design, 261
Research process, steps in, 262b
Research utilization, 256–257,
  266
  direct, 267
  indirect, 267
  persuasive, 267–268
  in practice, 267–268

validating study results in,
  266–267
Resource management, 304–305
Restricted-response questions, 69
Resume, experiential, 6–7
Reviewing past, 5–7
  experiential resume in, 6–7
Rights, patient's, 331–335
RN. *See* Registered Nurse (RN).
Rodgers, Martha E., 117
Role theory, 113
Root-cause analysis, 176–177
Roy, Calista, 117–118
Roy Model of Adaptation, 118

S
Sacrifice resolution, of conflict,
  241
Sample selection, in research, 263
Sample size, 263
Scanning, in reading, 62–63
Scheme, 5
Scope of practice, 110–111
  for Licensed Practical
    Nurse, 111
  for Registered Nurse, 111
Secondary health care, 296–298
  care management in, 298–300,
    299b
    cultural, 301–302
    developmental, 302
    social, 303
    spiritual, 300–301
  discharge planning in, 304–305
  outcome priorities of,
    297–298, 297b
  requirements of, 297
  resource management in,
    304–305